MANHOOD

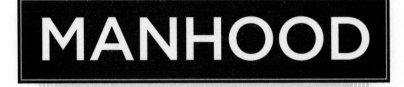

MANHOOD

HOW TO BE A BETTER MAN—

OR JUST LIVE WITH ONE

TERRY CREWS

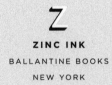

ZINC INK

BALLANTINE BOOKS

NEW YORK

While the events portrayed in this book are accurate to the author's recollection, a few of the names have changed.

Published in the United States by Zinc Ink,
an imprint of Random House, a division of Random House LLC,
a Penguin Random House Company, New York.

BALLANTINE and the HOUSE colophon are
registered trademarks of Random House LLC.
ZINC INK is a trademark of David Zinczenko.

ISBN 978-0-8041-7805-1
eBook ISBN 978-0-8041-7806-8

Printed in the United States of America on acid-free paper

www.ballantinebooks.com

2 4 6 8 9 7 5 3 1

FIRST EDITION

Book design by Casey Hampton

To the love of my life, Rebecca,
who taught me that I don't have to be perfect . . . just faithful

CONTENTS

PART 3
FALLING AWAKE // FAMILY

PROLOGUE

I HAVE TO PREFACE THIS BOOK WITH A STORY. IT WAS A blazing hot summer day in Southern California, the perfect moment to sit in an air-conditioned movie theater and relax with a wonderful, special effects–driven Hollywood extravaganza, expensive candy, crunchy popcorn, and an ice-cold drink. I had promised my seven-year-old son, Isaiah, that we'd do what we call "Man Time"—something very rare in our household, which is mainly comprised of the female energy of six women—my wife, four daughters, one granddaughter—and our twelve-year-old female house dog, Coffee.

Isaiah and I both agreed a movie would be the perfect respite from the heat. Being men, we decided our movie would be *Iron Man 3*. It being summer, there were product tie-ins for the film everywhere we looked, and I actually owned a fairly pristine original print copy of the third issue of the *Iron Man* comic book. So even though my son had never seen the first two movies in the franchise, he *had* to see the new one, and he was at the impressionable age where, if he didn't see *Iron Man 3,* he wasn't cool.

We found the perfect seats, sat down with our snacks, and endured what seemed like an hour of previews. Isaiah was noticeably wincing through most of them, but I attributed this to the fact that the movie theater had a really loud sound system. Then, finally, the movie started. Robert Downey Jr. was as compelling as ever, the effects were amazing, and the action was ramped up to eclipse the first two movies. I was enjoying myself.

Then I noticed something.

Isaiah's face was caught in a twisted frown, one hand in his popcorn, the other covering his eyes as he peered through his small fingers.

"Isaiah, you okay?" I asked, thinking maybe he had to go to the bathroom but didn't want to miss anything.

"Yeah . . . ," he said, his hand still stuck to his face.

I shrugged and turned back to the movie. A bomb exploded, and one of the bad guys appeared to die. I heard a whimper next to me. My son was gritting his teeth, holding a bunch of popcorn in a clenched, sweaty fist, paralyzed with his hand in the bag of popcorn. He was shaking.

"Isaiah, what's wrong?"

"Nothing. I'm okay."

But something was clearly not okay. More intense scenes occurred seconds later, and he tensed with every one. I knew I had to do something.

"Isaiah, let's go to the lobby for a sec."

He nodded, and we headed out into the lobby. Our eyes squinted as we adjusted to the sunlight and found a spot against a wall. I took a knee so I could examine his face as I talked to him.

"Isaiah, are you scared?" I asked, as gently as I could, so it wouldn't sound like a taunt.

"Uh, no. I'm okay." His face was still squinting, well after our eyes had already acclimated to the light in the lobby.

"Isaiah. It's okay. You can tell me. There's nothing wrong with being scared. Even Daddy gets scared sometimes. You can always tell me if you're scared. There's nothing wrong with that. Are you scared?"

"Yes . . . ," he said with a nod, appearing defeated.

"Isaiah, you wanna go home? We can get in the pool. Would you like that?"

His face relaxed and brightened, and I knew I had found the answer.

"Yeah! But the movie—"

"Don't worry about the movie, man. The most important thing is that we have Man Time."

I smiled, and he cheered up immediately.

"Isaiah, always tell me if you don't like something, or if you're scared of something. I'm not disappointed in you if you are, but I would be disappointed if you didn't tell me how you really feel. I love you, man."

"I love you, too, Dad. Let's go swimming!"

With that, we threw all of our concessions in the trash and headed out into the hot sun.

'D LOVE TO BE ABLE TO TELL YOU THAT I'VE ALWAYS BEEN like this: patient, caring, thoughtful, and a good listener. But the truth is, for most of my life, I was just the opposite. I was impatient, uncaring, hardheaded, and ignorant. I was selfish in every way possible, a brute to my wife, and a tyrant to my kids. My older daughters can tell you I've made them sit through movies they were scared of, just because they asked me to take them. *No pain, no gain. My way or the highway.* Right? Well, that's what I thought back then. I was the classic, type A, alpha male to the core. A strong, athletic competitor who used all of the charm and wit at my disposal to manipulate family, friends, coworkers, and everyone around me into giving me exactly what I wanted, and if they didn't, I was going to get them back one way or another.

I am a man. That's what men do. Kick ass. Take names. Do the job you've been paid to do. Accomplish your dream, no matter what it costs you or who gets hurt. He with the gold makes the rules. You crying? I'll give you something to cry about. That's life. That's the way it is.

I couldn't have been more wrong.

After we came home from the theater that summer day, I watched Isaiah run down from his room in his bathing suit and leap into the pool, as happy as I've ever seen him. I became overwhelmed with emotion when I thought about all of the wasted opportunities, the dumb mistakes, the ruined family trips, the things I should have said, and the hard lessons I'd had to learn in order to get to this place of greater clarity.

We absorb the world's lessons young: Be brave. Be tough. Show no weakness. Have no pity. Isaiah went to that ideal of manhood that day. He felt he needed to be tough for me. Endure this test for me. *I can do this.* Even when he couldn't. He denied how he felt, even as his world was crumbling all around him. Male pride is like walking a ledge on the side of a building, and any taunt or challenge will keep a man out there—until he falls to his death. I talked Isaiah down off that fictional ledge, at a movie theater. *At seven years old.* But now he's free. Until the next challenge.

I've been out there. I was on that ledge for more than forty-one years. Thinking that this is what manhood is. Being scared to death but never admitting it. Yelling and being angry with everyone, like I was holding on to the side of a building, because, psychologically, *I was*.

I've been searching my whole life, trying to find out what the definition of manhood is. Was it my father, Big Terry, when he went to work as a foreman at the GM plant in Flint, Michigan, with his work shirt ironed and his work shoes shined? Or was it Big Terry, drunk after work, and descending into the dark place where he made everyone in our household afraid? Was it Big Terry's calloused hands? His ability to build anything and everything? The fact that he put a roof over our heads and shoes on our feet? Was it the preacher who worked our church up into a frenzy of righteous fervor, rolling on the floor and speaking in tongues, but had dark secrets of his own? Was it five-year-old me, lifting our household furniture to feel strong? Or me, at age ten, starting my own secret life that would haunt me for the next three decades? Or me, finding football in junior high and being told by one miraculous coach that this could be my way out? Or me, getting married the day before my twenty-first birthday? Or me, being drafted into a seven-year career in the NFL? Or me, having been featured in more than forty movies and three hundred episodes of television, and earning success as a pitchman for three of the most popular brands in the world? Was any or all of that being a man? This book addresses that question—to both men *and* women—and explains, through the story of my life, what I've discovered. Welcome to *Manhood*.

MANHOOD

1

TRUE LIES

SPIRITUALITY

CHAPTER 1

SUPERHERO

I ALWAYS FELT LIKE A SUPERHERO. AND EVERY SUPER-hero has an origin story. The Hulk got hit with gamma rays, Batman became an orphan, and Spider-Man received that infamous bite from a radioactive spider. My origin story happened when I was two years old. My mother and father were arguing, a common occurrence in our cramped upstairs apartment on Albert Street in Flint, Michigan. An extension cord was plugged into the living room wall to power a nearby lamp. As they fought, I put one end of the cord in my mouth while it was still attached to the wall socket. It blew up, and I got shocked. My mother said I never made a sound. No screaming or crying, just a bloody, smoking lower lip with a hunk of skin hanging grotesquely from my chin. The cord at my feet told her what had happened.

Panicked I was in cardiac arrest—or worse—because of my eerie silence, they both rushed me off to the hospital. My mother was questioned by nurses, doctors, and even the police, as they harbored suspicions about her story, but eventually—to her great relief—child abuse was ruled out. A sense of gratitude accompanied the realization that it could have been much worse: I could have been electrocuted. Instead, the jolt of electricity gave me my "superpowers" and the scar I still have on my lower lip.

As I grew up, I loved hearing about my superhero beginnings, and I asked my parents to tell me the story again and again. As they told and retold it, I sometimes imagined I'd been electrocuted and had died in that room. I had visions of God sending angels to bring me back to life because God had determined I was special. Not only that, but I also saw God speaking as the doctors did in the opening titles of my favorite show, *The Six Million Dollar Man:* "I can rebuild him. Make him stronger." My imagination as a child stayed on overdrive at all times and has remained just as vivid to this day.

The matriarch of our family—my wise, tough-as-nails grand-aunt, Mama Z—put the piece of my lip in a mason jar and kept it on her mantel. Needless to say, my mother was horrified every time she saw it, as it had blackened into a tough jerky, and she was happy when Mama Z finally threw out her macabre souvenir. But for me, this family legend was just more proof that I was special. The story made me feel exceptionally tough because I'd survived something that should have killed me. My quarter-sized keloid scar on my bottom lip has always been a reminder of my strength and survival.

When I was three, the arguments with my father became so unbearable that my mother moved out of our Albert Street apartment and joined Mama Z and her husband, Brother Wright, on their farm just outside Flint. My mother, my older brother, Marcelle, and I lived in their attic for a year. I loved every minute of our time there, especially running outside among the chickens, pigs, and cornstalks.

Mama Z talked nonstop while Brother Wright sat in the kitchen nodding *yes* or shaking his head *no*. She was an amazing cook and prepared feasts, which I devoured. My hunger embarrassed my mother, and she always told me not to ask for anything. But she also told me not to lie. And Mama Z constantly asked me if I was hungry. I looked at my mother, noticed her angry squint, but still I nodded *yes*. Mama Z fixed me a huge plate of meat, beans, vegetables, and potatoes, as well as peach cobbler packed with ripe peaches she'd picked behind the house. I grinned at my mother until she reluctantly smiled back, knowing she'd been foiled again.

My mother often left us alone with Mama Z, a tough cookie who worked outside every day and introduced me to how real the world could be. In the morning, she stood in her kitchen, declaring there would be chicken for dinner as Brother Wright nodded in agreement. Then she went out back by the barn and looked for a good-sized chicken. I sat on the back stoop, watching as Mama Z tiptoed around with the fowl, almost mimicking their steps.

"Here, chickee, chickee, chickee," she called out in the sweetest little-old-lady voice imaginable.

Then she violently yanked the bird she wanted out of the crowd and held the neck still while spinning the body around in circles like a jump rope. When she let her victim go, the other chickens scattered and clucked loudly as her chicken—its neck broken, head dangling near its feet—ran around the yard flapping its wings for what was the longest minute of my short life. As the runaway chicken came near me, I recoiled on the stoop, scared to death it might attack me.

"Go on in the house," she said, waving me inside.

When she carried in the chicken, she promptly dunked it in boiling water, then plucked, gutted, butchered, and fried it. I watched every step, determined that I was never going to eat that bird. But as time went on, I grew hungrier and hungrier, and by the time she placed that same chicken down in front of me, with white rice and corn, I ate every bite. Plus seconds. It was the best chicken I ever tasted.

After a year with Mama Z, my mother and father reconciled, and we moved back in with my father. But not all reunions are happy. Before long, there were plenty of reasons I started feeling the need to be tough, even though I was only in kindergarten. We relocated to a small, ramshackle house on Flint Park Avenue. My father, Big Terry, began getting ready for the birth of my little sister, Michaell, and he and Trish, which is what we called my mother, moved Marcelle and me into the smaller of the two bedrooms.

At sixteen, my mother had given birth to my brother, and then had me at eighteen. I now suspect her youth had something to do with why we never called her Mom. And I believe we didn't refer to Big Terry as Dad in order to make it easier on Marcelle because he wasn't Marcelle's birth father. The fact that we had different fathers was never hidden from Marcelle and me, and I often wondered what Marcelle's father looked like and what he was doing. I thought about how it would feel to not know or have contact with my birth father, and I was always sensitive to what it must be like for Marcelle.

Once Big Terry and Trish had moved us into the smaller bedroom, they stacked our beds into bunk beds, which my brother and I loved because they now earned our highest compliment. "It's just like on TV!" we shouted when we ran into the room and saw them for the first time. I prowled around, trying out amazing feats of strength and showing off for Marcelle. Superhero-style, I lifted dressers and the living room couch and flexed endlessly, imagining electricity still running through my body. I would take the bottom bunk because I had a bad habit of falling out of bed in my sleep. I was also a bed wetter. Until I was fourteen.

Looking back on that time, I realize that my bed-wetting had something to do with how unsafe I sometimes felt in that house. One of the first nights my brother and I were sleeping in our new room, I woke up from a sound sleep to rumbling in the house that felt like thunder. *BOOM. BOOM. BOOM. BOOM. BOOM.* I lay in the dark, trying to make sense of where I was and what was happening. The whole place was shuddering. Trish was shrieking and screaming. It was pandemonium. I'd never heard anything like that before in our house, but nothing could have prepared me for those sounds anyhow. It felt like war.

Our bedroom door was closed, but light leaked in from the other side. My father had just installed a makeshift divider between our bedroom and the living room. It was uneven and allowed light and sounds to filter through the cracks to where we lay. I heard Big Terry's booming footsteps and a weird shuffling sound. It felt like an earthquake was shaking everything. I thought of my favorite Godzilla movies and wondered if the house would fall down like when he destroyed a city. I was scared of what was happening, and I stayed in my bed with the covers pulled up over my head. Marcelle did, too.

It became common for me to wake up to these sounds. And soon, there was a night when the chaos spilled into our room as my mother burst through the door.

"I'm going to take the boys and go," she said.

Big Terry followed close behind her. She had left before, and he knew she was serious. "Don't, Trish," he said, his voice pleading.

I blinked against the light, scared, trying not to do anything to make it worse.

"I'm telling you, I'm gonna take them," she said.

Something in Big Terry seemed to snap.

"You do that, and you'll be sorry," he said, his voice growing angry.

Trish yanked me out of bed and held me in her arms, gesturing toward the door. Big Terry's silhouette hulked over us in the darkness. He was yelling now.

"Calm down, Trish! Calm down."

She held me closer, my heart beating wildly, scared of what would happen. And then, just like that, she placed me back in bed. I pulled the covers up over me.

"Go to sleep!" she yelled at Marcelle and me.

Trish stormed out of the room, Big Terry close behind her. They slammed the door, but I could hear them continuing their argument in the living room. Sleep was impossible. My nerves were on high alert, and I stayed up for hours until the adrenaline finally wore off, and I fell into an uneasy sleep that left me exhausted.

Eventually, Marcelle and I grew bolder and climbed down out of our beds in our matching onesie pajamas to witness the action in the other room. I was the one to open our bedroom door so we could see what was happening, and we both peeked out. In the living room, Big Terry and Trish were fighting. Her hair was all messed up and crazy, and she looked like she'd already been hit a couple of times. She had something in her hand—a kitchen utensil, maybe.

"You ain't nothin'!" she screamed. "I'm sick of you. You're a drunk."

"Leave me alone!" he screamed back at her, slurring. "Leave me alone, Trish. Don't make me do something."

Marcelle and I stood there, wiping the sleep from our eyes, watching it all go down, wondering how it was going to end. She hit him, and when that didn't make an impact, she started pushing him.

"Don't make me do something!"

He pushed back, and she slipped a little, and then she hit him again.

"You made me do this!" He hauled off. *POW*. He hit her so hard she fell down and started crying. For a second, it all went quiet except for the sound of her sobs.

"I'm sorry," he said, leaning down toward her. "I'm sorry. I'm sorry."

"Get away from me!" she screamed. "I hate you! I hate you!"

These were our parents, and watching them fight was unreal. Big Terry was aptly named, as he seemed like a giant, his hands the size of bowling balls with calluses that looked impenetrable. His every step shook the foundation of the house, and his deep voice filled my little boy heart with fear. My mother was by no means a shrinking violet, though, and she could prod, taunt, and goad without mercy. She called him every name in the book, and I knew even then that a woman could cause violent pain to a man by lancing his pride with a few skillfully aimed obscenities.

Over time, as these fights kept repeating themselves night after night, Marcelle and I started treating them like scenes in a movie. As the shouting and shoving started, he hopped down from the top bunk.

"I got Trish," he said, already moving to open the door.

"Okay, I got Big Terry," I said. "Who's gonna win?"

"I don't know," he said.

We weren't being cold or unfeeling. We were just trying to cope with what we couldn't understand, and maybe even put a cheery face on a dark moment. The fact that two people who said they were in love—our parents—could hurt each other so much was too difficult to comprehend.

I threw off my blankets and followed Marcelle out into the arch of the living room doorway. Trish pushed Big Terry, and he pushed her back. They were grappling, both trying to get a grip on each other, almost like wrestlers.

Marcelle and I giggled. "Get 'em, get 'em," we whispered to each other.

We were trying to make this nightly horror into a fun game, hoping the violence would finally stop, and we could be a family, just like on TV. Big Terry pulled back and punched Trish. She went down. We immediately stopped giggling. It wasn't a game. She was lying on the floor shaking. It was an awful thing to see my mother in pain, and to have my father be the one who had hurt her, but I didn't feel safe enough to go over and check on her.

I imagined being punched like that and wondered if I could take it. Was I strong enough? When I considered how large and strong Big Terry was, I knew that even this superhero was no match for that supervillain disguised as my father.

"I'm sorry," Big Terry said.

Even though his voice had grown softer, Trish drew back from him.

"Get away from me!" she yelled. "You hit me. You hit me."

This is not on TV, I thought. *This is not the way it's supposed to be.*

Unless.

Is this what all men do? Is this what the families on TV are like when no one is watching?

I couldn't believe it was true. I felt so helpless. I couldn't stop Big Terry. I couldn't save Trish. I couldn't do anything. Where was the electricity I should be able to summon when I needed it, at times like this? I balled up my tiny fists, but there was nothing there. I was little, weak, and scared. I needed more strength, more power, more courage. I could only watch and hope that the violence stopped, wishing someone would take me away from all of this. Trish looked up and saw us standing there. "Go back to bed," she said.

When we didn't move, she sternly repeated herself: "Go back to bed!"

We knew she would turn right around on us, and we didn't want her wrath or one of her legendary whuppings, but we paused before going back to our room.

On other nights, when Big Terry was the first one to notice us, it was a different story. "Go back to bed," he said.

Although that's what Trish usually wanted, when *he* said it, she flipped.

"No, they need to see you hit me," she said. Even when she was in pain, she took revenge on him with continued attacks on his pride.

We froze in the doorway, wanting to make it better, or at least not make it worse. She looked back at where we were huddled together. I stood a little in front of my brother, trying to shield him, although he was two years older than me. He'd just been held back a year in school, and I felt like I had to protect him. In fact, I felt like I was there to protect everybody. That's what superheroes did.

"No, you all stay right here," she said to us. "You see him?"

Even at five, I knew this was wrong. We were being used to hurt Big Terry. I didn't want to be a pawn in this cruel game. I looked over at Marcelle. He was crying. Then I broke. I started to cry, too. As young as I was, I still felt mad at myself for not being able to keep my emotions in check, like I'd done when I'd been shocked.

"See, see what you did to them!" Trish said to Big Terry.

He turned and stormed out the door. She lay there on the floor, weeping. Marcelle looked at me. I nodded at him and led the way back to our room. I heard Marcelle shifting in his bed above me, and then he grew still as he fell asleep. I stared at that top bunk for hours, waiting to crash out, or for the sun to rise, jumpy with adrenaline as I relived the fight scene again and again.

We had this little cassette tape player back then. Trish didn't normally let us listen to secular music. It was either gospel or no music at all. But there was one folk pop group, The Free Design, that she tolerated. They had a breezy, harmless little tune called "Kites Are Fun," which I probably heard a million times as a kid. It was the kind of song that made it impossible to remain in a bad mood. When I was wide awake and all twisted up after one of their fights, I closed my eyes and sang it again and again, trying to get the visions of what I'd just seen out of my head. Kicking my imagination into overdrive again, I formed a visual of Big Terry, Trish, Marcelle, and me, all flying a kite. I desperately wanted that image to come true. Finally, I fell asleep. When morning arrived, I usually woke up in a wet bed.

Since I couldn't fly away from our problems like a kite, I decided I would work even harder to be strong like a superhero. I ran around the house, lifting one end of the couch, and then the other, as if my superpowers were about to kick in. The fabric was yellow with a black paisley design, and I used to fight it as if it were a vicious lion. You know, ghetto games. From the couch, I raced over to the gigantic entertainment console, an enormous solid block of wood and metal that looked like a brown refrigerator lying on its side. The radio was on one end, the record player on the other. On top, my mother kept a heart-shaped box given to her by Big Terry. Its Valentine's Day chocolates long gone, it remained, a symbol of many things. Although the furniture was impossibly heavy, I'd grab one side and heave it up, just to see how far I could lift it into the air. Something about the voluntary stress and strain of lifting things made my brain calm down. I needed to move things. It was my way of feeling like I was taking control of my situation.

It didn't take long for me to end up with a sharp pain in my side. When it didn't go away, Trish took me to the doctor. I'd given myself a hernia. I was five.

As I was pushed down the hallway of Hurley Medical Center on a gurney, I watched the holiday decorations slide by on the walls, and the ceiling tiles pass by above me. I was a kindergartener with a Technicolor imagination, and Christmas was a big deal. Every song, image, or decorated tree had a seasonal story. Even though I was in the hospital, I was happy. I felt special because I was getting extra attention.

I was so small, and everything seemed so big. A man put a plastic mask over my face, and I looked around—like, *what?*— until the anesthesia pulled me under. I was afraid I was going to feel the surgery, but when I opened my eyes again, the procedure was over. It seemed like I'd closed my eyes for only a second and then magically moved from the hallway to a bed in a hospital room in the kids' ward.

The room smelled familiar, like our kitchen, with its scent of food and Pine-Sol. Toys were scattered on the ground, but I was feeling weird, and in no mood to play. I looked around and saw

I was trapped in a giant crib, its jail-like bars encircling my bed. There was another little boy in a bed across the room near the window. He kept talking and talking and talking. I wanted him to stop, but he wouldn't. Finally, I couldn't stand it.

"Hey," I said.

He just kept right on chattering away. I looked around. Trish was very strict, not only about the music we listened to, but also how we behaved. I wasn't allowed to swear at all, and even "shut up" was considered a cuss. I didn't see anyone.

"Hey . . . shut up," I said.

For a moment, I experienced the rush of having broken the rules. It felt good to be bad, even if it was only for a second.

"Who are you talking to?" Big Terry's voice grumbled down from above me.

I was lucky that I was already stretched out, because I had a baby heart attack. I knew I shouldn't have said it. I was generally a good kid who didn't break the rules, and not only because I didn't want to get caught. I really wanted to be good. Here it was, the one time I'd dared to disobey, and now I was going to get it.

I can't get away with anything, I thought.

But Big Terry started to laugh. I don't know if it was because Trish wasn't around, or because he felt bad I was in pain. He was much more patient with me while I was in the hospital. Up until then, the entire experience had been overwhelming and scary, but now I saw that maybe it had an upside, too. Not to mention that I got to roll Big Wheels in the halls during the week I recovered.

AS FRIGHTENING AS MY SURGERY HAD BEEN, IT DIDN'T lessen my attempts to prove how strong I could be. One of my earliest memories of my sister, Michaell, who we called Micki, happened a few years later when she was just learning to walk. I was hanging out on our front porch, showing off for my friends from next door.

"Look, babies are really strong," I said.

I held out a stick and had Micki put her hands on it. And then I lifted her up.

"Look," I said.

Of course, I wasn't really showing them how strong babies were. I was showing them how strong *I* was. And as I found out, babies really aren't that strong. As soon as she was in the air, *WHOOSH,* she lost her grip and, *BAM,* she hit the ground and started screaming. *Oohh,* I thought, already knowing what came next.

Trish ran out and swooped up Micki, who was still crying.

"What are you doing?" Trish glared at me. "What happened to her?"

"She fell," I said, backing away. "She fell."

I admit it, I lied right to Trish's face. I lied so quickly, even though I knew it was wrong. I wanted to be a good kid, but I had a greater desire not to get a whupping in front of my friends.

That day, I got off easy. But more often, I did not. When things were good, Trish was very playful and sweet, but when things weren't—and often, they were not—my mother could be extremely cruel. Like the time I yanked the buttons off my new coat, just because I couldn't believe how easy it was to pull them off, or how magical it felt: the gentle *POP* sound, and the feeling of the smooth round disc in my hand. And then another *POP,* and I'd pulled the next one off, too. Trish saw me sitting there with the buttons in my hand and snapped. I scrambled to my feet.

"Aaaah," I screamed, running around the house, trying to escape her.

If we had to get a spanking, we always hoped it would be from Big Terry. He never hit us, and he probably only spanked me twice in my entire childhood. He knew Trish would kill him if he put his hands on us. One time he spanked Marcelle a little too hard and left a welt, and Trish just flew at him. He never did that again.

Trish caught me. She always did. She bent me over, pulled her arm back and brought the belt down. Hard. *WHAP*. It hurt, and I screamed in earnest now.

"Be quiet," she said.

She hit me again, harder, which only made me scream louder.

"I said shut up," she said, hitting me again.

It didn't correlate. She was hitting me with a belt and expecting me to remain quiet. I forced myself to stay silent, hoping it would be over sooner if I did what she said, but the whuppings were always long, and drawn out, and horrible. It felt the same way it did when Big Terry and Trish were arguing, and it started to get nasty and violent. I could see her go into a zone, as if it wasn't about my brother and me anymore, but some war she was having with Big Terry, and Flint, and herself. Looking back, I think there were times she was just so mad she couldn't help herself. She was mad at herself for having us so young, for not being able to live the way she wanted and for being trapped in her marriage with us kids. Her behavior was also the result of her upbringing. Her mother was very cruel to her, and that's how the cycle goes until someone stops it, like my siblings and I have done with our kids.

CHAPTER 2

IS THAT WHAT A MAN IS?

WAS ALWAYS WATCHING BIG TERRY, WONDERING: *IS that what a man is? Is that what I'll be like when I grow up?* It was tricky, though, because he was two different people, and I was never sure which one was going to show up around the house on any given day: Big Terry on his way to work or Big Terry on his time off.

My father was talented with his hands and a very hard worker. He was a foreman at the GM plant in Flint, where he worked the second shift. And so I always watched him leave for work in the afternoons, but I rarely saw him come home. Day after day, I had a visual of my father going one way: out the door. When I woke up in the morning, he was usually asleep. We weren't supposed to disturb him, but of course we always did. I mostly just wanted to peek in and look at him because he worked a lot, and he slept a lot, and I didn't get to see him much.

As quietly as I could, I tiptoed over to their room, opened the

door, and just stood there, watching Big Terry sleep, a sheet
pulled up over his chest. I was filled with wonder and awe. My
father had muscles and was strong. He had huge hands and feet,
and they were so rough. I wanted calloused hands like that,
hands that seemed capable of doing anything. A loud snore
erupted from him, making him sound like a monster, and he
rolled over but didn't wake up.

Is that's what I'm going to be like? I wondered. I shut the door
gently and hurried back to my room before I did anything to get
myself in trouble.

I always knew as soon as Big Terry woke up because I could
hear him. *BOOM, BOOM, BOOM, BOOM.* "Trish, Trisha!" he
yelled as he came into the kitchen.

I was sitting with Marcelle at Big Terry's latest creation, a
wooden diner booth, which we loved because it made the
kitchen resemble a real restaurant. Trish was making Big Terry's
dinner, beans cooked with oxtail, which he ate at noon before
work.

Wow, that's how I've got to walk, I thought. I wanted to be big
and strong just like that. I wanted to be able to make things like
the wooden clock Big Terry was carrying, which was lined with
velvet and could really keep time.

"You made that?" I asked.

"Yeah, I'm going to sell these," he said. "We built the pyra-
mids, boy! You know that, right?"

I sure did. This was his favorite saying. I nodded my head at
him.

"That's how I know we can build anything else, too," he
said.

I nodded again. Just from watching my dad, I learned that if
you want more, you have to do more. I know I got my work
ethic from him.

Big Terry had enlisted in the Army right after high school, and he always dressed with the extreme precision of a soldier. He was big on clothes.

"If you look like a clown, they're going to treat you like a clown," he often said. "But when you look like a man, you'll always get treated like a man."

For work, he wore an impeccably ironed shirt with a pocket protector for his pens. When we got older he made us iron everything we wore, even our jeans and T-shirts. He was a stickler for shiny shoes, too, and he always put care into polishing his own. I used to sit and watch him getting ready for work, wanting to be close to him and learn about the ways of the world from him. He held a black leather work shoe in one hand and drew a soft rag over its toe with the other.

"So you got black polish for those?" I asked, hoping to draw him out.

"Yep."

He kept on buffing. When he was on his way to work, all I could get out of him were these clipped, one-word answers. Still, I hung around, hoping for just a little more from him. But he was in a hurry, and before I knew it, he was out the door.

Marcelle and I learned how to stay out of Trish's way, and we were happy playing together around the house when Big Terry was at work or out. I could draw for hours, lost in sketches and crayon drawings of people, monsters, and muscled heroes. I'd started drawing when Marcelle was in kindergarten and I was home alone with Trish. To keep me busy, she set out crayons and pencils on our brown wooden coffee table, and I knelt over the blank paper. She grabbed a pencil with her left hand and showed me how to make a few shapes to get me started. I, too, grabbed the pencil with my left hand, and then my imagination took over.

When I finished a picture and held it up, she was obviously impressed. Now, this is the thing: I've always been hooked on praise, so when she told me that my drawings were really good, I took to it just like that. I felt like I needed to increase the acceptance and admiration I received around the house because, most of the time, the climate was just the opposite. Drawing was cathartic. I could visualize a different kind of world and control what happened there, at least in my pictures.

I loved to draw but quickly learned there's nothing that comes naturally to us. We may have interests and desires, but we still have to work hard to improve our abilities. I drew all of the time, and I enjoyed it, but I also found it extremely frustrating. Trish and Marcelle would praise a picture, and I'd be happy with it. But then I would go to sleep, and when I woke up and looked at the same picture, I saw it as a mess. It was a constant fight, trying to get what I visualized to match what I put down on paper. Finally, the struggle became part of the process for me.

Whenever we heard Big Terry's car pull up outside of our house, Marcelle and I packed up our fun. We knew to be wary of the person he usually was outside of work. *BOOM. BOOM. BOOM. BOOM.* He banged into the living room, unsteady on his feet, and leaned against the wall, scowling at us. Too late. I was trapped.

"I told you to do the grass," he said.

Marcelle and I looked at each other and headed upstairs to our room without saying anything. We knew he wouldn't hurt us, but he had a way of making things so uncomfortable when he was drinking that we didn't want to be around him.

I didn't have to be downstairs to know what came next. Big Terry had a regular routine. He went over to the stereo console and put on his favorite record, Bobby Womack's soulful anthem to lost love, "Woman's Gotta Have It," and played it as loud as he could. If I passed through the living room later in the night, it was hard to even look at him. He'd gone to work neat as a soldier. Now he was collapsed in a heap, a beer in one hand. His hair was mussed, his T-shirt wrinkled and stained. Usually he wanted to be alone in these moments and did his best to ignore us. But there was no way to ignore him, sitting there crying to himself and playing his music. Finally, Trish couldn't take it anymore, and she stormed into the room.

"Why are you here?" she said. "Why don't you go somewhere with all that?"

I agreed with her, but I held my breath, hoping he wouldn't suddenly snap and yell or hit her. He was pulled up too far inside of himself to lash out.

"Ugh, you're messing with my time," she said as she walked away.

All I ever wanted from the pre-work Big Terry was for him to slow down long enough to talk to me. But usually, only the drunken Big Terry felt like talking, and I didn't want to be around him. I didn't know what to make of the things he told me. All of the secrets from his childhood came spilling out, as he described being raised by his grandmother in Edison, Georgia, and how he never knew his father, and his mother lived down the street, but she didn't want anything to do with him.

"My mama didn't love me," he said. "Your mama loves you."

I couldn't understand it at the time, but I always felt like he was envious of Marcelle and me. And he made it abundantly clear that, by his standards, we had nothing to complain about. He judged the love he showed us by what he did for us. His attitude was always: *You guys are eating. You guys have clothes. You're lucky.*

"You have it good," he said to us, again and again.

Whenever Big Terry got going like this, I tried to hide out in my room. But when he'd been drinking and wanted to talk, he came barging in, flipped on the light, and held court. I startled awake and lay in my bed, blinking against the glare, scared because he was big and loud, even though he wasn't yelling.

"Boy, I love your mother," he said, looking at me.

I just stared back at him, paralyzed. He came closer to the bed.

"I love you guys," he said to Marcelle and me, standing by our bunks.

In spite of everything, I puffed up with happiness. This was all I really wanted from him, and I was still smiling when he stumbled out of the room and downstairs.

Not long after that, Big Terry was leaning over a square of newspaper, shining his shoes before work. I strolled up to where he sat and smiled at him.

"Hey, I love you," I said.

"Mm-hm," he said, not even looking up.

It was like the moment when he'd been a loving dad had never happened. I was crushed.

Even though I didn't like being around Big Terry when he was drunk, I wanted so badly to connect with him that I went into the living room one night when he was in his chair, beer in hand, listening to Bobby Womack. I leaned in and kissed him on his cheek. He looked at me like I was crazy. I backed away from him so quickly I nearly tripped over my own feet, and I never made that mistake again. Whether he was sober or drunk, I kept myself apart from him as much as I could.

THE ONE PERSON I COULD COUNT ON WAS MY BROTHER, Marcelle. We were always paired together. We shared the same socks and underwear and wore the same outfits in different colors, and we were often asked if we were twins, even though we looked nothing alike, and we couldn't have been more different. Marcelle was very small and handsome, with lighter skin and softer hair. I was the spitting image of my father and earned the nickname Little Terry. My mother had this sing-song way of calling out each of our names around the house: "Mar-SA-yell! Lil TER-REE!"

Marcelle and I traded comic books, ripping out the ads in the back for books by the first great bodybuilder, Joe Weider. We also loved anything Bruce Lee. He had his own fitness regime, and we ordered his books to learn all about it. From him, we began to understand how to use one muscle against the other, like by pushing our hands together as hard as we could.

I was obsessed with constantly making myself bigger and tougher. I was always thinking about which moves I could do while I was watching TV, and I flexed my legs so hard in the shower that my muscles cramped. Trish thought I was crazy, but the really wild thing was how well it worked. I grew notice-ably stronger.

Being big and strong meant everything to me. Even though I was the younger brother, I continued to feel like my family's protector. If someone said something to Marcelle, I was the one to respond. But then there was the day when an older guy came up on Marcelle as we walked home from school. I started de-fending my brother. And then I stopped short. *That guy's too big,* I thought. *I can't do anything.* The kid attacked Marcelle, beat him up, and threw him in a rosebush. *Ow.* When the bully was gone, I held out my hand to Marcelle and helped him to stand.

"Man, you didn't even have my back," he said.

"I'm sorry. He was too big. I didn't know what I was going to do."

Marcelle accepted my apology, but Trish did not. She was furious at me.

"Don't you ever, ever let him get beat up," she said. "You take care of him."

Because Marcelle had been diagnosed with a learning disability and held back a year in school, we all felt the need to take care of him. But Marcelle was determined to prove he wasn't dumb. I often came into our room and found him reading the dictionary, trying to learn a new word every day. His quiet determination and commitment to self-improvement left a big impression on me.

I had my own reason to worry people might think I was stupid. I was in the kitchen with Trish one day when she said something, but I couldn't make it out.

"Huh?" I said. "What?"

"You can't hear me?" she asked.

I shrugged, not wanting to get in trouble.

There was no hiding the problem, though, and finally, my mother and father took me to a specialist at the University of Michigan in Ann Arbor. After we'd gone through all of the tests, the doctor said my hearing was fine and sent us home. But still, there were times when I missed something I was told to do at school or around the house because I hadn't heard the person speaking to me. We went to another specialist, and again we were sent home. By the third or fourth doctor visit, Trish had had enough. Before we even got out to the car, she started in on me.

"You know what?" she said. "I'm not taking you to any more of these. You take those tests. And they say nothing's wrong. Is there something wrong with you?"

"No," I said. My big thing was I didn't want to get held back. I'd seen what it had done to my brother, and I was determined it wasn't going to happen to me. I didn't want anyone to think I was dumb, either.

When we were in the car on our way home, they were sitting in the front seat, and I was alone in back. Trish suddenly whipped around and looked at me. I realized she'd been talking to me, but I hadn't been able to hear her.

"Huh, what'd you say?" I asked.

"There ain't nothing wrong," she said. "You're faking it for attention."

"No, he ain't faking it," Big Terry said. "There's something wrong with him, Trish. He don't know what you said."

My father's sympathy meant a lot to me, but Trish was done. My mother was very conscious of her time, and as far as she was concerned, I'd wasted enough of it.

And so I did learn to fake it: hearing, that is. As a kid, I pretended to hear whole conversations that I couldn't really make out, smiling and nodding along with the others. I soon learned to mirror faces. If two people were talking, and one person said something that made the other person laugh, I laughed, too.

And that's how I got by. A few years ago, I finally acknowledged that getting by was not the same as being able to hear, and I went to another specialist. I learned that my hearing is fine, except within a specific decibel range, like the high-pitched voice belonging to a woman or child, and then it's gone. Even so, as the specialist said a series of words to me, I was able to repeat them back to her. And then she covered her mouth and asked me to repeat what she said. I couldn't do it.

"Your whole life you've been reading lips," she said.

"Are you serious?" I asked.

I had no idea because I'd developed so many work-arounds by that point. When I started acting, I memorized everyone's lines, so even if I couldn't understand the words the other actors

were saying, I could tell where in the conversation my lines were
meant to be and say them at the right moment. And always, I
mirrored others nonverbally with my face, which I'm sure was
actually one of the most helpful skills I could have acquired as
an actor. Back then, I was just learning to pretend.

Even more than I wanted to prove I wasn't slow, I wanted to
show everyone that I was a good kid. Like most children of al-
coholics, I was a pleaser. If something would bring peace to the
house, I'd do it. I never really shared what I wanted, because
nothing I wanted was as important as keeping things calm.

I also wanted to be right for God. When I was little, we attended the Church of God in Christ, which had a way of driving
home the importance of being virtuous and the terrifying consequences of the alternative. It helped that I've always had a big
imagination and could see further than the present moment,
which meant I had a clear sense of the consequences of my actions, even when I was little. Being left-handed and right-
brained, I've since learned that, scientifically, I have a tendency
toward imagination rather than analysis, and that's absolutely
correct.

On Sundays, we went to church from eleven to four, and
then we returned for night services, from seven to ten. One day,
when I was in the first or second grade, I just couldn't take it
anymore, and I fell asleep during the day service. I woke up
groggy, already worrying that Trish would be mad at me. And
then I sat up quickly, a much deeper fear spiking my heart. My
mother wasn't sitting next to me, and neither was Marcelle or
Micki. There was no one in the pews. Everyone was gone.

It was my worst nightmare come true, the one our pastor
and Trish had warned me about time and time again, the one I'd
worried about at night in my bed. It had always been preached
to me in our church that God was coming, and if I was in sin at

the exact moment he arrived, then he would take all of the Christians with him, and he would leave me behind. It was a horrifying thought. I could never commit a sin, because I didn't know when he would appear on earth, and I didn't want the moment of sin and the moment of reckoning to be the same. But now it had happened to me. The Rapture had come, and I'd been left behind. *What did I do?* I worried. I'd obviously committed a sin, but I had no idea what it was.

I was too petrified to move, and I sat in that pew, my heart knocking in my chest. And then I heard a noise from the rear of the church. Slowly, fear tingling throughout my body, I crept back toward the stairs that led down to the basement. The sound of voices floated up to where I stood, but that didn't reassure me at all. Who knew what tortures awaited me and the other sinners who'd been left behind down in the church basement? By the time I got downstairs, I was crying. I recognized the faces I saw. They were people from our church. But I couldn't stop.

"Where's my mother?" I said. "They're all gone."

"No, no, no, we're here," Trish said.

I ran to her and threw myself into her arms. I was so relieved. They'd gone downstairs to have dinner and left me upstairs to finish my nap without thinking anything about it. I'd been spared that day, but the depth of the fear I'd felt when I thought I'd been left behind only strengthened my devotion to being good. I'd always been an antsy kid, and that episode heightened my nervousness and increased my desire to be as perfect as possible.

In layman's terms, members of the Church of God in Christ denomination were Holy Rollers. Our pastor started out services very steady and deliberate, kind of like a train pulling out of the station. Slowly but surely, he ramped up his talk into a feverish, singsongy yell, punctuated by whooping sounds, as if he were clearing his throat. I was told that, if a preacher never reached this point in his sermon, it was considered a waste of our time.

"Oooh, he sho did preach toDAY!" the women of the church said at the end of each successful service.

But, as far as I could tell, no one could ever decipher what the service was about. When the preacher started "whooping," the music minister jumped on the organ and added musical exclamation points. As the mood grew loud and emotional, people in the congregation began to scream and jump. Sometimes while the preacher paused between shouts, the music took off, and people ran around the church in a delirious haze. One lady sprinted from the back of the church, down the center aisle, and slammed full force into the communion table. She fell to the ground writhing as the "mothers" of the church—older women who were the female counterparts to deacons—draped sheets over any body parts exposed as the result of her "receiving the spirit." As a child, watching grown men and women turn into wild people who sometimes frothed at the mouth was more than a little upsetting.

To the church, people had one of two spirits: the Holy Ghost, or the spirit of Satan. I wanted no part of anything Satanic, and so I wanted to "receive the spirit," in order to ensure I was right with God. I began to ask people how I could make it happen. No one could tell me how. My mother told me it was a feeling deep inside, and others said it would just overtake me. I prayed and prayed. At every church service, I waited for this thing that would come and take me, making me run around, shaking uncontrollably, and speaking in other tongues. But it didn't happen.

During one of these manic services, our preacher proudly surveyed the spiritual ecstasy set to music. "If you don't feel nothing . . . then you must not HAVE NOTHING!" he exclaimed, smirking righteously for effect.

I was crushed. I felt nothing, so . . .

I couldn't believe it. Just then, my friend JoNathan Watkins, who was sitting next to me, leaped to his feet and started shouting and jumping. JoNathan was one of my few good friends at the church, a kid my age who was in the same situation as me: trapped at services most of the time. We'd hit it off by joking while the preacher spoke, and soon developed complex games to pass the time, all while appearing to be interested by what the Elder was saying. Any ill-timed giggle, outburst, or horseplay would bring down the wrath of our mothers or other church-goers, and the certainty of a whupping for me at home. We grew skilled at being the good little boys who always appeared respectful, while making slick fun of the church's authority figures when they turned around.

I looked at JoNathan, waiting for him to signal to me that this was a ploy—just another game he'd invented to make the long church service pass a little faster. But he was giving me no such signs. He kept shouting, hopping, and speaking strange words, over and over again. I couldn't understand what was happening.

Oh, NO! I thought. *The spirit skipped right over me and got into him! What am I not doing right?*

At first I thought I'd been passed over because I'd been jimmying the channels on the cable box just right so the adult channel, Escapade, came through. But no, JoNathan had done that, too. *How come he got the Holy Ghost and not me?* I was sad and confused. I felt like God didn't deem me worthy, so I had no choice but to get worthy and become a person God paid attention to, before it was too late.

It wasn't just because of the scare tactics employed by our church that I maintained a deep, personal faith. I knew God loved me, and I felt protected by him. I knew that we have to be good to others. I didn't want to be a jerk. I wanted good things to happen to me. In order for this to be possible, I tried to be a good kid.

But because I was a pleaser, it wasn't enough to be a good kid. I had to be the best kid ever. I became almost like our church's poster child. While many kids in the church were necking in the bathroom, smoking cigarettes and weed, and doing all kinds of forbidden stuff, I was the opposite of that. I was there for every service and youth group session, and I always volunteered for everything.

The pastor leaned into the pulpit. "Who wants to say the prayer?" he asked.

I raised my hand. As I looked around, I realized my hand was the only one aloft in the entire congregation. It looked like I was saying the prayer.

"Who wants to sing? We need someone to solo in the children's choir."

Again, my hand was the only one in the air.

It reached the point that our youth minister would come to me when she needed a volunteer from the congregation. She knew I'd always say yes, and that I would do whatever I'd been asked to do perfectly, so I'd make the church look good. And I always did. Because I was such a pleaser, I was always down to do whatever I was asked. I also knew it was a way to make my mother like me, to make people in our church like me, and to make God like me. And that was all I wanted. I lived so much of my life scared, and I really wanted to please God so he would protect me and take care of me. I also had a very long-term mind-set about who I wanted to be, and I didn't want any bad decisions I made now to catch up with me later in life.

When I was in the fourth grade, I started playing the flute during our church services. It was Mama Z's idea to give us instruments.

"Baby, what instrument do you want?" she asked.

I considered my options. The only musician I knew was my Uncle John. He was a cool guy, a jazzman, and he played flute and saxophone. I decided I would play flute, too. Marcelle asked for a guitar. I didn't grasp the significance of this conversation, or think about it again, until the following Christmas. Underneath the tree was a guitar for Marcelle and a flute for me, compliments of Mama Z. As soon as I saw Marcelle's guitar, I realized I'd made a huge mistake. I should have asked for a drum kit. But it was already too late. I was a flutist.

For the next four years, once a week, I went over to John's house every Wednesday after school for my flute lesson. On top of that, Trish made me practice for an hour every day. Soon enough, I was a pretty good flute player. And so it wasn't long before they recruited me to start playing the flute in church at the Sunday service. So there I was, in my little red suit and my big black Afro, standing in front of the congregation, playing along with the organ. While we played, people kept jumping up to holler and scream, but I kept playing, and Trish and our pastor beamed at me. I felt a moment of peace. I was a good kid.

CHAPTER 3

DOUBLE LIFE

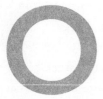UR CHURCH FELT PEOPLE WERE BEING TOO worldly if they listened to secular music, wore makeup, went to dance clubs, played sports, or went to the movies. *The Exorcist* was huge around that time, and our church used its success to prove "the devil" was in the country's movie theaters. The only thing that was permitted was to eat, and there were more obese people at our church than in all of New Orleans.

I didn't like these rules, but I mostly got along fine. It helped that Big Terry once broke ranks and took Marcelle and me to see *The Apple Dumpling Gang,* although he snored through the whole thing. Now, whenever I nod off during a movie with my kids, it cracks me up. We really do become our parents. Also, although we couldn't go to the movies, when a film was shown on TV, we could see it. I always thought this was strange, but no one could ever give me an explanation.

Trish was a big television fan. Marcelle and I were allowed to have a television in our room from my third-grade year, when we moved into our house on Winona Street, until we grew up and moved out. On hot summer nights, Marcelle and I watched TV with a fan blowing on us, drinking cold Kool-Aid and eating Paramount potato chips and bologna sandwiches with mustard, followed by glazed crullers from Dawn Donuts down the street, until Trish commanded us to bed. We watched all of the prime-time shows, including *Good Times, The Jeffersons,* and *Sanford and Son.* And then, on Saturday nights, we watched *The Love Boat.* African-American kids didn't have many role models on TV at that time, and Isaac on *The Love Boat* was our guy, as were the characters on the predominantly black sitcoms. We really held on to them. It was like, *Wow, maybe we are just like on TV. Maybe we're actually worth something.*

Marcelle and I playacted out the scenes we'd just seen, faking heart attacks and get-rich-quick schemes, and singing, "If I didn't care . . ." with candy rings on our pinkie fingers. Anytime anyone did something stupid—except for Trish, of course—we borrowed the line from *Sanford and Son* and said, "You big dummy."

My favorite character was also from *Sanford and Son.* Aunt Esther, played by LaWanda Page, as a bible-toting, gospel-preaching, purse-swinging crusader who suffered no fools. This character reminded me of so many women I grew up with that I thought the writers must have gone to our church.

I actually got much of my sense of comedy from TV, but from a source that might surprise you. It wasn't Richard Pryor, even though I loved him, too, and faithfully watched all four episodes of *The Richard Pryor Show.* It was Carol Burnett. *The Carol Burnett Show* was my absolute favorite. She didn't care about being cute—even though she was—because she was so committed to her comedy. She could sing, dance, and tell a joke. I was in awe of her, and she still means a great deal to me.

So even though I felt like I was missing out when the other kids at school talked about some movie they'd seen, I had plenty to keep me entertained at home. And then, in 1977, a few months before my ninth birthday, I was exposed to something for the first time that impacted my life in the most profound way possible: *Star Wars*. This was different. Even though movie trailers back then never actually gave away what the movie was about, we knew from the television commercials that this was the best movie ever.

Marcelle and I didn't dare ask Trish, but we were desperate to go. And then we experienced the kind of miracle I could believe in: Aunt Paulette asked if she could take us to see *Star Wars* at the drive-in. Marcelle and I begged and begged for Trish to let us go. I think we would've collapsed into a heap and never recovered if she denied us, and Trish knew it. Finally, after a long protest, she acquiesced. We couldn't believe it! We were going to a real movie at a real drive-in movie theater!

Marcelle and I were ecstatic as we piled into Aunt Paulette's purple Pontiac Monte Carlo with the landau top and drove to the Miracle Twin Drive-in Theater in Burton, a suburb of Flint. When the sun set, the whole parking lot buzzed with excitement. This was more than a movie. This was an event. I was so glad to be a part of it. The John Williams score hit, and the *Star Wars* logo snatched me into its vortex. For the next 125 minutes I was so enthralled I couldn't move. It was like I was actually there among the aliens, warriors, and Stormtroopers.

It was as thrilling as any experience I'd ever had. In fact, that movie changed everything. Immediately, I knew this was what I wanted to do. It never occurred to me to be an actor. But I was definitely going to make movies someday. I was an artist, so I figured I could be an animator or a special-effects person. But first I had to get out of Flint. And I had no idea how I was going to do that.

THERE WAS A MUCH MORE SERIOUS CONSEQUENCE OF attending a church that strict. It was an open secret that many people in our congregation led double lives. We knew it was happening all around us, but we never talked about it. There were known homosexuals who sang in the choir but chose to keep their lifestyle quiet to retain their membership. There were men who had second families across town. And it was later revealed that our pastor was using cocaine, frequenting prostitutes, and even attempting to sell drugs while still preaching.

Because I saw supposedly virtuous adults behaving in these ways, I believed a hidden, subterranean life was normal, and my own secret side bloomed around this time. When I was nine, I was at my Uncle John's house for my flute lesson one day when I went down to the basement to play. In one corner, not even all that hidden, I came across a bunch of pornographic movies and magazines. At first I just stared at the images of naked women in disbelief. I knew it was wrong. But I was already excited. Even though it was bad—or maybe because it was bad—I was tempted to look, just like JoNathan and I did with the Escapade channel. I opened a magazine and examined a picture. I was too young to do more than stare, but I liked how it made me feel. I got a rush from doing something I wasn't supposed to do.

And then, suddenly, I was afraid. I threw down the magazine and looked up quickly. The basement was empty. No one had seen me. But God had seen me. If he'd come down to earth at just that moment, I would have been left behind for sure. I had to pray to be forgiven and swear never to look again. I ran back upstairs feeling nervous and uncomfortable, hoping if I kept my promise I'd avoid getting in trouble.

WANTED SO MUCH MORE. I HATED THE DRINKING AND STU-pidity I saw around me. The divide between all I wanted for myself and the limitations of my surroundings pressed down upon me. There was Uncle Jesse, who drank so much he developed gout and lost both his legs. And still, he got us kids to bring him drinks in his wheelchair, even though he was already slurring so badly he could hardly speak.

My step-grandfather, William, who once told my mother I was the ugliest baby he'd ever seen, put on overalls every Saturday and detailed his Cadillac for hours, paying more attention and care to that car than he ever did to his own family. When finished, he dressed up and rode around in that highly polished car until early Sunday morning, leaving my grandmother at home.

Even my own father had a double life. We sometimes received strange calls at our house from some woman telling Trish what her husband was up to on the side.

"Who are you?" Trish hissed into the phone. "Leave us alone. You're gonna have to bring that up with him. I don't care."

She slammed the phone down. But she couldn't make it go away.

Another time, Marcelle and I were standing in front of the church with Trish when some lady came up to us from out of the crowd. She scowled at Trish.

"You know your husband ain't no good, right?" she said.

The three of us stood together, glaring back at her until she was gone.

"What was that?" I asked Trish.

"Nothing," she said.

Big Terry had too much silence about everything, and he wouldn't talk about anything. He just got drunk, and cried, and listened to his records.

"Man, I messed up," he said.

We knew he was making penance somehow, but we never knew for what. I didn't want to be like any of these examples, but they were the men I saw around me. So if I wasn't going to be like them, how was I going to be?

I tried to glean information about the other men in my family. The stories were colorful, but not very clear. The only photo I ever saw of my paternal grandfather, James Crews, was a mug shot from when he was arrested for drunk driving. He had died in a car crash, which was all I knew of him, and I never met him.

On my mother's side of the family, my grandfather, General Simpson, and his brothers, Buddy and Arthur, were not to be played with. My great-uncle Arthur had quite the reputation. A very handsome man, he had ladies of all kinds competing for his attention. One time, he was having an affair with a man's wife. When the husband found out, he beat his wayward spouse. Arthur then went over to the man's house, beat him up in front of his wife, and told him if he ever put his hands on her again he'd kill him. The man never touched his wife again.

Arthur was not the subservient black man, either. When he lived in Florida, a white man once threatened him. He knocked the guy out cold in the street and was promptly arrested. This not being the first time he'd behaved in this way, a mob of concerned white citizens formed outside the jail. A police officer sympathetic to Arthur's plight sneaked him out the back door to safety. Arthur quickly made his way to Flint, knowing that if he stayed down south, his days on earth were numbered.

My Uncle Buddy had the biggest biceps I'd ever seen. He had a job cleaning and servicing planes at the Tampa airport, and his arms were unbelievably huge. He often flexed his biceps and asked Marcelle and me to try to make it go down. We punched, squeezed, even hung on it, but it was no use. It was like hanging on a tree branch. I wanted to be that strong, and I also wanted to be as funny and personable as my Uncle Buddy. But for all the fun he was, he also had a flip side. He'd been known to yank a man out of his seat with one arm just for looking at him wrong, and it was understood that many a man had been on the wrong side of his punches. But he was my uncle, and he loved me, and I always saw his good side.

My grandfather, General Simpson, lived in a small house on the outskirts of Flint. He and my grandmother, Mama, had been married for a few years when my mother and Aunt Paulette were born, but they divorced soon after. He worked in a fish market and had a gentle toughness about him that I loved. He was never harsh with Marcelle or me. When he smiled, wrinkles formed at the corners of his eyes, making them sparkle. It took a while, but I now see the same wrinkles around my own eyes when I smile. When we were small, he picked Marcelle and me up in his long, boxy Buick, a toothpick pointing to and fro in his mouth as he worked it around in his cheek, and a tan straw fedora slightly askew on his head with a small feather in its band. He took us to his latest girlfriend's house, and we hung out with their family until it was time for us to go. Not a lot of conversation, or a buckled seat belt on any of these trips, just an appreciation for the fact that he actually wanted to spend time with us. He was lonely, and I'd like to think having us with him helped.

My grandmother, Mama, later bought the duplex next door to my family's house as an income property. General had become very sick, and my mother was the only one looking after him, so he moved into one of the two apartments. One day, he and my Aunt Paulette got into a heated argument about how he was not there for them when she was a little girl. He tried to defend himself, but she hauled off and slapped him across the face as hard as she could. Everyone stopped and stared. He held his face and looked at her incredulously, then silently walked out the door.

To this day, the memory of that scene hurts me. Maybe he had not been the best father, but I had never seen him be violent or abusive to anyone, and even my grandmother never told tales of domestic violence or abuse. In fact, he still loved her, and often told her so when she visited him on his deathbed.

T HE TRUTH WAS, I WAS MORE LIKE THE MEN IN MY FAMILY than I would have cared to admit. It was definitely difficult to be good all of the time. When I felt anxious, my thoughts whipped back to the moment I'd stood in my Uncle John's basement, and how the pictures I'd found there had pushed everything else out of my mind. When it was time for my flute lesson, I snuck down into his basement again and again. I still wanted very much to be the good kid at church, and to be right with God, but I was soon creeping away to look at pornography whenever I could.

When Trish and I ran errands, I told her I was going to the drugstore to look at comic books, but I knew they kept copies of *Playboy* and *Penthouse* out with the rest of the magazines, and I stood there and flipped through the images for as long as I could get away with it. More than once my reverie was interrupted by a familiar scolding voice, and my blood seemed to freeze in my veins.

"Boy, I sent you in here to get something for me," Trish said. "And you're looking at that stuff?"

I quickly tossed the magazine back on the shelf and pretended I had no idea what she was talking about. She never really disciplined me because, to do so, she would have had to acknowledge the content I'd been exposed to, and she wasn't about to sit down and have a real conversation with Marcelle and me about sex or anything else. Plus, it would have been impossible for her to restrict our lives much more than she already did. We couldn't watch secular movies in theaters or listen to secular music, and we were forbidden to date or go to dances. And by that point, my interest in pornography went way beyond just a passing curiosity. The next opportunity I had, I snuck back into the drugstore. And I found other ways to see such images.

Ever since JoNathan and I had learned how to fix the cable box so the adult channel, Escapade, came through, we looked at it every chance we got. I'd seen pornography before, but this was the first time I'd viewed pornographic movies, and they captivated me completely. Looking back, I can see why. Not only were they full of sex, which thrilled me, but also, most of them were warped versions of children's stories: *Jack and Jill, Alice in Wonderland, Goldilocks*. Here we were, two "saved" kids, sneaking peeps at adult movies in between church services. Guilt made me think twice, but I'd soon figured out that our cable box at home worked the same way.

Marcelle and I were in our room one afternoon when we

heard Trish leave the house. As soon as her car door slammed outside and the engine noise grew faint, I looked up from my comic book to where Marcelle was studying on his bed.

In unison, we both jumped up and hurried into our parents' bedroom, where they had a cable box on their TV. I quickly moved the channel indicator up to the right spot, my heart beating fast, even though I knew Trish would be gone for at least an hour, and there was no real danger of getting caught. As soon as I found the sweet spot, an image of two naked bodies moving together on a bed came into view. I felt all of the tension within me release.

I soon established a pattern where, anytime I was dealing with anxiety, I acted out with pornography. On the one hand, I felt bad because I knew I shouldn't do so, but at the same time, it was exhilarating, a rush, like taking a drug. And it was a way to rebel against my incredibly strict mother.

Once I had access to pornography in our house, that's when it first became a problem for me. I watched it every chance I got. Marcelle watched it, too. Until the day he came into the living room, caught sight of the TV, and stopped short.

"Man, I'm not doing that anymore," he said. "I don't need it."

I stared at him for a long moment. I knew I should stop, too. But I couldn't.

"Shoot, you can go ahead," I said. "I'm gonna watch."

I felt guilty as he went upstairs without me, but I didn't turn it off.

And then, one afternoon when I was about twelve, I was sitting on the couch alone, watching the Escapade channel, when I heard a noise behind me. Trish had crept downstairs and snuck up behind me.

"What are you doing?" she asked.

I looked back and forth between her furious expression and the screen.

"Oh my God, what are you watching?" she said, her voice growing more and more agitated as she realized what was on the screen. "What are you watching?"

I was half standing, wanting to cover the image, turn the channel. She reached the TV first and snapped it off. We stood facing each other awkwardly. I knew I was in trouble. I was embarrassed, and I was scared she was going to flip.

She looked at me closely, as if she was trying to read my expression.

"Have you been . . . ?"

I stared at her blankly. I was so naive I had no idea what she meant.

"I don't know," I said. I wasn't lying. I really didn't know.

"Have you been, you know, masturbating?" she said. "You have, because you've been looking at that stuff."

"I don't know what you're talking about," I said. "I've never done that before."

I was like: *You can do that?* Then I started doing it. And sneaking even more porn.

My new habit was also a part of my ongoing attempt to figure out what it meant to be a man. There was no conversation about anything in our household, certainly not the birds and the bees, and so I picked up what information I could wherever I could find it. I was constantly wondering: *What does it take to be a man? When can I be called a man? Who's going to say I'm a man?* I became consumed by such questions, and I was on a quest to answer them for myself: *Is it being able to beat somebody up? Is it being able to drive a car? Is it a first kiss? Is it having sex?*

At the same time, my desire to be good became a quest to be

so perfect that I could make up for the bad things I did in secret. I was the primo yes man. And I was soon obsessed with achieving perfection in all areas of my life. This meant working harder, working more, becoming fitter, improving my art ability. It wasn't enough to paint a picture that my teacher and classmates admired. I had to paint the perfect picture. It wasn't enough to be good at sports. I had to be the best player ever.

The neighborhood I grew up in became worse and worse over the years, and when we played football in the street, or in a park, a handful of grown men always sauntered over to get in on the game. Maybe they were just reliving their youth, but they felt it was their job to make us tough, and they did not mess around.

I took my position, ready to get moving as soon as the play started. A big, grizzled man in his late twenties or early thirties, his arms roped with muscle, hunched down across from me, staring me down, psyching me out.

"Hey," he said. "You ain't gonna do nothin' in here."

As soon as the action was under way, he lunged toward me. I knew better than to show any fear. I ran at him just as hard as he was coming at me. With a whack that reverberated throughout my core, he smacked me down to the uneven asphalt. I lay with gravel poking into the back of my head, trying to catch my breath. In an instant I was up. If I showed any weakness I was done. We took hits that hard from grown men every time we played. It was really kill or be killed. Looking back, it seems crazy. I'd never let my son be in a situation like that. But I can tell you this: I became a better player. It hurt too much not to learn to run faster, get out of the way quicker, and take on full-body blows, all without complaint. As long as those guys were looking on, when we got hit, we brushed ourselves off and kept on going.

We had to decide whether we were going to grow up quickly, and be strong, maybe even earn enough respect from the older guys to make a name for ourselves, or if we were going to sneak away. A lot of the other boys my age knew it wasn't for them, and it didn't take them long to stop messing with these pickup games. But I wasn't going to show any fear. I was obsessed with my own internal mantra: *I'm big enough. I'm strong enough. I'm fast enough. Even if you beat me today, I'm coming back tomorrow.* That's how I first realized the power of physical fitness and athleticism, which soon took on an even greater significance in my life.

CHAPTER 4

A WAY OUT

ASKETBALL WAS THE FAVORED SPORT IN MY hometown, and I started playing in sixth grade. Pickup games in the summer were huge, and during Flint's cold winters, it was also a social thing, as well as a sport you could excel at indoors. In ninth grade I added football and track to become a consistent year-round athlete. I knew, however, I was not good enough at basketball to go pro or even play at the college level. Because there were so many great basketball players in the city who were better than me, I decided football would be my ticket out of Flint. My need to be the best meant that I not only threw myself into practice and did extra drills on my own time, but I also volunteered for everything. No matter what the coaches asked us to do, I was the first person to raise my hand.

Fortunately, during my seventh-grade year, I finally came under the leadership of a man who recognized not only how

hard I was pushing myself but also saw something special in me.
My football coach, Lee Williams, took an interest in me like no
one else ever had, and he became a father figure to me. His encouragement was crucial, arriving at a moment in my life when
it was enough to change everything for me going forward.

My father hated sports. He was all about the Army and
wanted me to enlist as soon as I graduated from high school. I
knew this was one of the only ways to escape Flint, and the only
way out that would also earn Big Terry's respect. But something
about this path didn't sit right with me. It wasn't what I wanted.

I was an artist, and now I was an athlete. I didn't know what
this meant for my future. But Coach Lee did. After yet another
practice when I'd worked as hard as if we'd been playing a
championship game, he pulled me aside. My first instinct was
always to fear I was in trouble, even though I didn't think I'd
done anything wrong.

"Terry Crews, let me tell you something," he said. "There's
no way you should not be playing football at a Division One
college on a Division One scholarship."

His voice was so sure and strong it was as if he was giving a
speech about me.

"Really?" I said.

"Terry Crews, you've got everything," he said. "There's
nothing you can't do. I see these other kids doing it at these big
schools. You've got all those traits right here. I see them. You can
do all that."

"Really?" I said again, too stunned to say anything more.

At first, I couldn't process what he was telling me. I drank in
his praise like a thirsty man. No one had ever encouraged me
like that before. It was all I needed.

I always tell everybody: All a kid needs is one good word

from someone he believes. It's not necessary to have anything more than that.

Coach Lee literally changed my life forever. And he was only my coach for three years. After my ninth-grade football season, another coach forced him out, which was devastating for me. But it didn't really matter by that point. Even after he was gone, I held on to his words forever. He had said I should be playing football on a Division One scholarship, and that was what I was going to do. As far as I could tell, it was going to be the best way to get out of Flint. It was perfect for me. I wanted to be strong. I wanted to be athletic. I wanted to be a superhero. Who's closer to that than an NFL star? I began to see myself as a football player.

Of course, not everyone else in my life was as supportive of my hopes and dreams, and not all of the experiences I had were so positive. As soon as Marcelle and I were old enough, Big Terry had us working every weekend, and all summer long, shoveling snow in the winter and mowing lawns in the summer. We hated it, but not because we had to work hard. I didn't mind making an effort when it came to painting, or lifting weights, or doing football drills. I resented the fact that Big Terry dropped us off and left us out there all day. Sometimes we did two or three lawns, and then, even after we were done, we had to wait for him to come pick us up. By the time he finally showed up, our whole Saturday was gone, and I was fuming.

The people we did work for gave our wages to Big Terry, and Marcelle and I never saw any of that money. So we had worked all day for nothing, not one single cent. As far as Big Terry was concerned, this was part of our lesson.

"I'm teaching you what it's all about," he said. "This is what it is."

Well, my takeaway from that was: *What's the use? Why bother working hard if you're not going to see any benefit from your endeavors?* It was clear to me from that moment on: If I was going to be working, I needed to be working at something I enjoyed. I made a promise to myself at a young age that I would always love what I do. Now, that's a wonderful, noble philosophy to live by, but it got me into some trouble down the line. When you're coming up in the world, sometimes you've got to do things you don't enjoy. Good luck telling my thirteen-year-old self that, though.

Anytime Marcelle and I did get a little bit of money, we had very different approaches to our finances. If I had five dollars, I went to McDonald's, and just like that, it was gone. On the other hand, Marcelle squirreled his money away under his mattress. I was a big spender. He was a big saver.

But then, without fail, Big Terry always came into our room at some point and stood there swaying in the doorway, looking back and forth between us.

"You guys got any money?" he asked.

"Nope, I spent mine," I said.

I looked at Marcelle, waiting to see what he'd do, knowing it would probably be better for him to lie and say he didn't have any money, either. But he couldn't lie. Even though it was obvious how badly it was tearing him up, he nodded his head.

"I got some," Marcelle said.

"Let me see it," Big Terry said.

Marcelle went over to his bed and pulled out his money. I'd watched him be disciplined for weeks and weeks, going without the treats I indulged in, until he'd saved a couple hundred dollars. Just like that, Big Terry held the bills in his hand.

"I'll give it back to you," Big Terry said.

Marcelle nodded at him, even though we all knew that was

a lie. Big Terry never paid him back, and he never stopped taking Marcelle's money. And so I learned another lesson from Big
Terry early on: If you work hard and save your money, somebody is going to come in and take it, so you might as well spend
it all.

B Y THE TIME I WAS IN HIGH SCHOOL, I'D HAD ENOUGH. I
was getting out, and that was that. With Coach Lee gone,
I started looking around for anyone else who might help me in
my goals, or at least support my dreams. Things had gotten beyond weird at our old church, and we'd finally convinced Trish
to join a new congregation. I had high hopes from the beginning. Our old church had been a whole lot of shouting loud and
saying nothing, whereas our new pastor was more of a teacher. I
decided I needed to have a meeting with him to talk about my
life and my plans for the future. We met in his office one day
after school. I got right to the point.

"Pastor Brown, I want to play football," I said. "I want to be
a football player."

"Oh, no, no, no," he said. "Football, that's not good. That's
evil."

"Wait a minute, you play basketball on Friday nights," I said.

"We play basketball at the church," he said. "But, in basketball, we're just trying to get a ball in the hoop. Football, you're
intentionally trying to hurt people."

I'd spent my whole life trying to be good, except for my one
secret habit, which I swore I'd never do again. And now, my
pastor was telling me that my ticket out of Flint was evil. I was
devastated and collapsed inside. He had no idea that, for me,
this conversation meant everything. He just kept shaking his
head.

"Yep, basketball is cool," he said. "Football, I would never recommend that."

I knew I wasn't intentionally trying to hurt anybody when I was playing. I was just trying to tackle them. I was just trying to be a good athlete.

That day changed everything for me. I still went to church with Trish and Marcelle, but I was hatching a plan in my mind.

I've got to leave, I thought. *I've got to get out of here. I've got to get a new life. There has to be more for me than these true lies I'm hearing.*

It was easy enough for me to bide my time at church, but it wasn't so easy at home. Trish and I didn't agree on anything, and neither of us was quiet about it.

"You hate me," she said. "I don't know what your problem is."

Well, there was our crazy church, for starters. And then there was the fact that she wouldn't let me date. Here I was, fourteen, fifteen years old, and of course I had an interest in girls, but she shut it right down.

"No," she said.

"Why can't I?" I asked. "Why can't I just go on a date or something?"

"Because you're stupid," she said.

I rolled my eyes at her and that just made her gain steam.

"Yeah, you're stupid," she said. "You're going to get somebody pregnant."

She was afraid, because she'd gotten pregnant at sixteen, and again at eighteen, before she was ever married. She saw Marcelle and me as little boys still, and she was sure the girls out there were going to take advantage of us and tie us down. She didn't know that she was a lesson for me of all I didn't want my life to be.

——

A S THE EIGHTIES PROGRESSED, THE CONDITIONS IN FLINT grew more and more dire, and I became more and more determined to get out by any means necessary. All of the auto plants were closing. People were getting evicted and leaving town. Schools were shutting down. Homes were falling empty and becoming increasingly decrepit. Then the crack epidemic hit. With the drugs came more violence. Every time there was an event in the neighborhood, people got shot. Let me tell you, I lived *Roger & Me*. Whenever someone asks me about where I grew up, I tell them to watch that movie. That's exactly what my high school experience was like.

Our school was a magnet school that bussed kids in from all over, so it was 60 percent black, 39 percent white, and 1 percent other minorities. We were located right in the middle of the roughest neighborhood in the city, and gang members and drug dealers often hung around the building, waiting to put any egghead black kid or scared white boy in their rightful place.

Once I was leaving basketball practice when this thug we all knew as Julio took my shoe from my gym bag and ran outside. I chased after him but stopped short, almost needing a diaper, when I saw notorious Flint drug dealer Donald "Juice" Williams and his gang sitting astride their customized Chevrolet Chevettes.

"What you gon' do?" Julio taunted me.

Knowing I had to maintain a strong appearance, I didn't show my fear.

"You better give me my shoe back!" I said, trying to sound tough.

"Come get it!" he said, looking to the gang with him, showing that he knew, that I knew, that I didn't have a chance.

"Give the kid his shoe back," Juice exclaimed.

So Julio threw it back. It landed about five feet in front of me. I grabbed it and quickly found a ride home, my nerves frayed by thoughts of what almost was.

FROM TENTH GRADE ON, I WANTED OUT OF FLINT SO BADLY that playing football well enough to earn a scholarship became my sole obsession. Trish continued to forbid me to date, but I'd decided I didn't want a girlfriend anyhow. I didn't want anything that would tie me down. It was fine to like a girl from afar, but that was it. Nothing was more important to me than my ticket out of town, and I couldn't lose focus.

Luckily, around the time I lost Coach Lee, I made friends with a kid named Darwin Hall, and he became that one person I needed to help me believe in my dreams. In eighth grade, I'd tried to steal one of his French fries. He hit my hand and then got into a karate pose. Rumor had it he was a really good martial artist, and so I made nice, and we've been best friends ever since. That's how guys meet: a challenge is thrown down, and then with mutual respect, a friendship can grow.

In tenth grade, Darwin transferred from Flint Academy to another high school, but I still went over to his house almost every day. I felt guilty for leaving Marcelle stuck at home, but I was at an age when I needed to carve out my own life for myself. Darwin had five sisters, all much older than him, and his parents mostly left him alone, so we often had his house to ourselves. We spent most of our time in his basement without adult supervision. We were well aware of the possibilities.

"We could be doing all kinds of things," I said.

"We could be smoking weed," he said.

"We could be having girls."

"But we've gotta be good if we're gonna get anywhere."

And we were. Instead of going wild, we just hung out to-gether, watching movies, listening to music, break dancing, and getting real with each other.

"Let's talk about what we're gonna do," I said. "Let's talk about the future."

Darwin was a computer geek, so we talked about that, even though there were times it made my eyes glaze over. And we talked about my two great loves—football and movies—even though neither really interested him. We talked about what we wanted our lives to be like, where we would live, and what kind of women we would marry. Most important, we made a deal that whenever one of us learned something—about girls, or school, or life—we would always tell the other person.

My dad certainly wasn't teaching me anything. In fact, he was always telling me to do something he'd never explained to me before—like the time he made me change the oil in my mother's car—and then, when I did it wrong, he got mad at me. That hurt me badly. I didn't understand how he could expect me to know something I'd never been taught. It seemed more and more like the adults in our lives couldn't be trusted, and we had to figure out everything for ourselves. We pulled away from our parents and spent most of our time together, looking ahead to a future when we'd be free. Trish was not happy about this.

"You always want to go over to his house," she said. "You always want to be away from us. What's your problem?"

"I just, you know, I'm not dating, I'm not doing anything," I said.

But even the innocent activities we were getting up to were enough to upset Trish. It was no secret that I've always loved to dance, and on Saturdays and Sundays, Darwin and I practiced break dancing for, literally, twelve hours straight. We worked out routines and went over them again and again, until we were as perfect and synchronized as we could be.

Now, here's the thing I really couldn't understand. Trish loved to see me dance. When we were at family dinners she was always making a big deal about it. I was fooling around in the kitchen, popping in time to the beat in my head, when she pulled me out into the living room, where everyone else was visiting after dinner.

"Ooh, show the family that one move you're doing," she said.

Let's just say I've never minded being the center of attention, so when Trish said dance, I danced. I lifted my arms and re-created the move I'd just shown her.

"Aw, that's so cool," Trish said.

She smiled at me, and she seemed softer somehow. Even though I knew the answer she'd given me so many times before, I figured it couldn't hurt to ask again.

"Okay, can I go to the dance, then?"

She wasn't smiling now.

"No, you're not allowed to go to dances."

That just crushed me, after I'd spent so many hours practicing, and she'd even made me dance and complimented me in front of everyone. So that's how I came to do the worst thing I ever did as a teenager—well, besides my double life.

I told Trish I was staying over at Darwin's house, which, technically, I was. As soon as I got over there, I put on my gray and red Puma track suit. And he put on his black and red gear. We warmed up a little bit in his basement, and then we snuck out and picked up Carlos, the third member of our dance crew, and went to the dance in my high school's gym. I know, bad boys, right?

Trish truly had nothing to worry about. Going to these

dances wasn't about girls for me. I hadn't even slow-danced with a girl at that point. It wasn't about the hip-hop, either, which of course she couldn't tolerate one bit. It was about getting on the floor, and finally enjoying the payoff for all of the hard work we'd done in Darwin's basement, by showing off all of the stuff we could do.

There we were, in the regular high school gym where I played basketball during the week, but with the beat pumping and the lights flashing, it felt like a real hot spot. Well, okay, almost. I looked at Darwin, and he looked at me, and we started doing our thing. Almost instantly, everybody circled up, and they flipped. With my classmates screaming and hollering, the adrenaline hit, and I was in bliss.

When we went back to Darwin's house later in the night, I was on a high.

I loved performing, and I knew I wanted to work in entertainment, once I'd used football to get me out of Flint. I begged Trish to let me dance in the school talent show, but she was not having it. I couldn't reconcile how big my dreams were with how small she forced my life to be. I racked my brain for a compromise.

"Can I host the talent show, then?" I asked.

She looked at me hard, as if she was trying to search out the sin in this.

"Well, okay," she said.

I got to host the talent show, and at least that was something. But I couldn't line up her rules, which seemed so arbitrary to me, with my behavior, which I knew was good overall. Well, except for my one secret, and I was always swearing I was going to give that up forever. So I couldn't keep my mouth shut about what I saw as the injustice of her rule, given the fact that I had no interest in going out and being the reckless idiot she accused me of wanting to be. This meant that Trish and I fought constantly. I was so sick of living at home by the time I was a teenager, and during my last few years of high school, that our relationship ground to a halt.

Even though I was a varsity athlete who played football and lifted weights—and I mean I'd gotten big by this point—Trish often got physical with me. When she was mad, she slapped Marcelle and me like it was nothing, as if we were still little kids. Usually I didn't let it get to me. But one time I said something, and she whacked me. Before I could stop myself, I lifted my hand in the air, just as a reflex.

"You raise your hand at me?" she snapped.

There was no way I was really going to hit her, and I was already lowering my hand. But Big Terry happened to come into the room just then.

"Ugh, leave me alone," I said and started to walk away.

Trish turned from me to Big Terry with a wild look in her eye.

"Terry, he was gonna hit me," she said. "He was gonna hit me!"

I was already on my way up the stairs, but my father started running after me. He couldn't reach me on the stair above him, so he tried to kick me. The next thing I knew, he was screaming. I looked back, totally confused. He'd kicked me in the butt, but it hadn't hurt at all. Well, he'd chipped a bone in his foot. Served him right.

I left Big Terry on the stairs, screaming, and went into my room and shut the door.

Taking my place at what had become my regular spot, I stared out the window into the street. There was nothing to see, really, but at least it was a reminder that there was a whole world out there. *I've got to get out of here,* I thought.

Of course we weren't allowed to buy any secular music, but I loved rap music, and I had a little boom box. I sat there at the window for hours, recording snippets of whatever songs I could catch on the radio. My favorite song was "Sucker M.C.'s" by Run-DMC, and I often managed to record part of it, but for some reason, I could never catch the entire song on the radio. Even just hearing part of it was something, though. The music, the view of the street outside, I held on to these and whatever other lifelines I could find for myself. It was a hard time.

No matter how wrong I believed my mother to be during those years, I can look back now and see that she was doing the best she could. Even though I wanted to be good, it was far too easy to be in the wrong place at the wrong time in Flint during the eighties. And I really didn't get that. I was young. If there was a shooting, my mentality was: *Yeah, but I didn't get shot. I'm fine.* Trish was trying to keep us from getting hurt. She was trying to keep us from slipping through the cracks like so many other young men around us did. So many guys I knew from that time have gone on to have six kids by six different women, or ended up in jail. Or ended up dead.

Darwin was the only person I felt like I could really talk to, and our long conversations about our future plans were another lifeline for me. But even he didn't know my darkest secret. Sure, there were times we got a porno tape and watched it, but it was almost like sex ed, just trying to figure out what was what.

"Is this how it goes down?" he asked.

"I guess," I said. "Is that what I have to do there?"

We craned our necks and studied the screen.

In spite of Trish's obsessive fear that Marcelle or I would actually be around a girl long enough to get her pregnant, like had happened to her when she was our age, she never educated us about how to prevent this, except to once ask us if we knew how babies were made. I had many questions, but I was way too squeamish to talk about it with her. And while it would have been better to have a conversation about sex with Big Terry, of course he never talked with us about anything.

Sometimes when Darwin and I saw porn, I wanted to come off as a good guy.

"Man, don't look at that," I said. "We don't need that."

He was cool with this and had no reason to suspect I was watching pornography at other times, so he didn't know the extent of my obsession. No one did. My secret was safe. But I knew I was doing it. I knew it was wrong. I felt bad. And yet I couldn't stop. And so my hidden life started to chip away at me, little by little. After I had binged, I clasped my hands over my chest at night, listening to Marcelle sleeping in his bed across the room, and I prayed so hard to be good.

"God forgive me, please, please," I said. "I'm sorry. I'll never do it again."

There were times when I abstained for a month, or two months. And then I always slipped. After a while, I figured this was just how my life was going to be, and that it must be normal. Everyone must have a double life like I did.

CHAPTER 5

TAKING MY SHOT

THE ADULTS WE WERE SUPPOSED TO LOOK UP TO and respect didn't seem to be living any better than I was, really. There was a substitute teacher in my high school who knew I wanted to play football at a Division One college and then play in the NFL. He had attended the University of Michigan, which has one of the best teams in college football. One day in tenth grade, he pulled me aside.

"I went to the University of Michigan," he said. "You've never been to a University of Michigan game. You won't believe it. It's incredible. You'll love it."

I was excited just thinking about it. What a cool guy he was to invite me.

"Wow, okay."

Soon after that, this substitute teacher picked me up at my house on a Saturday morning. I couldn't believe I was going to a University of Michigan game. The whole drive down to Ann Arbor, he talked up the experience.

"Man, I love this," I said. "I want to go to the University of Michigan."

He looked at me out of the corner of his eye as he drove.

"Terry, now, you know you probably can't go to the University of Michigan."

All of a sudden, what he was saying made me feel sick.

"Well, why not?" I said.

"Michigan is another animal," he said. "I mean, it's just—the competition is huge. You want to go where you could really thrive."

For the rest of the day, I didn't hear another word he said. He took me around and introduced me to all of his fellow alumni, and he brought me into the stadium where 105,000 people were screaming for the game. He was cheering and yelling himself. But it all meant nothing to me. *What good is it being here?* I thought. *You're showing me something you're saying I can never have. What in the world is wrong with you? You're going to take a poor kid, show him a feast, and say, "You can never have it. No, no, no, the dog food is for you. This, however, is how the nice guys live."*

I looked around the stadium, and I was sure everyone could see I wasn't good enough to be there. It was a very long day. When he finally dropped me off at home, I didn't thank him, and I never, ever talked to him again.

Luckily for me, I didn't accept his words. Instead, I got mad. I knew I was good enough to make something out of my life. But how many young people believe the limiting things they're told? That's why we've got to define our circumstances for ourselves. I'm telling you, our sense of ourselves is all we have in this world.

Even though I knew who I was and where I was going, I had to fight hard to hold on to this knowledge, because high school was full of such experiences. In twelfth grade, I had this basketball coach who felt like he could do no wrong. I mean his ego was just out of control.

We had a star player on our team, Craig Sutters. Now, the problem wasn't with Craig. He was one of the most gifted athletes I've ever seen. He could literally take a quarter off the top of the backboard. I mean, this kid could jump. He could throw. He could shoot. He was a superstar. All of us players, we loved Craig. Because he was such a good guy, and we were so glad he was on our team. The problem was what the coach had to say about Craig in relation to the rest of the team.

One day after school, we were sweating our way through practice. I took a shot, and I missed. The coach blew his whistle and stopped the action on the court.

"Terry!" he yelled. "Terry, what's wrong with you? You think you can shoot better than Craig?"

"Ah, I mean, no, but I had an open shot, so I took it."

"You know what? Here," the coach said, throwing me the ball. "Shoot the ball. Shoot the ball. You think you're better than Craig. Shoot the ball."

Practice was completely stopped. I was stuck out there in front of everyone. It was incredibly embarrassing. So I shot the ball. Of course, I missed.

"See, you'll never be as good as Craig. Never. Don't you ever shoot the ball again. You pass it to Craig. That's what you do."

Well, I got the message. He had designated shooters, and that's the way he wanted us to play. So that's the way we played. No matter what I did, I felt like this guy hated me, but I never gave up. And he didn't have a better athlete to put out on the court, so he had to play me. Anytime I had a shot, I passed to Craig.

That year we were the team to beat, and we went all the way. Finally, we made it to the last championship game. Well, the other team, Flint Hamady, used this technique where they kept passing the ball back and forth without making a play, in order to run down the clock. My teammates and I wanted to attack, but Coach was having none of it. We did as we were told and sat back, but Coach was clearly choking. At the end of the game, we managed to score a shot, which left us within two points of victory, with five seconds left on the clock.

The other team threw the ball into play. I made my move, and I stole it. I took the ball the whole length of the court until I was right under our basket, and then I looked around. Craig was all the way down in the corner. Even if I passed to him, there was no way he could score.

FIVE. FOUR. THREE.

I did a layup.

TWO.

The ball rolled onto the side of the basket. And then it fell off.

ONE.

The buzzer sounded, and the place went nuts. Hamady had won, and it was a huge upset. They stormed the court. Everybody on our team collapsed. This was our senior year. Craig wasn't coming back. I wasn't coming back.

We went into the locker room and sat around, waiting for our final talk from Coach. He came in and stood in front of us, clipboard in hand.

"I want to thank you guys for your effort this year," he said.

"Now, if Terry had thrown the ball to the right guy, Craig was right there under the basket."

Not only was this untrue, but even if his fantasy was the reality, what then? We would have had a tie? Maybe? Craig still would have had to make the basket.

Hey, wait, I thought. *We were losing. I stole the ball. If the guy had just held on to it, we would have lost anyway. There were five seconds left.*

He'd painted it like I'd cost us the game, and I couldn't figure out why. It wasn't like we were winning. We'd already lost. My attempt was a last-ditch effort.

"Terry should have thrown the ball to Craig," Coach said. "But that's the way the world works. Some people don't make the right moves. And we all have to pay."

That was a major moment for me. Coach was someone I'd been told to follow. And his words simply weren't true. It was yet another occasion when I realized I couldn't always listen to adults. Sometimes they didn't make sense.

The aftermath of our defeat was even worse. The next day the local paper ran a story that basically said: "Terry Crews had the last shot. He missed."

One of my teammates believed Coach, and he called me out at school.

"Man, you should have passed the ball to Craig," he said.

I looked at him. Hard. "What did you say to me?"

"Everybody knows you should have passed the ball. You cost us the game."

"Dude, leave me alone."

He got up in my face. I wasn't having it. I hit him right in the mouth. *POW.*

He fell to the ground. As he scrambled up and away from

me, I looked down the hallway and locked eyes with the hall guard.

"Terry, I saw the whole thing," the guard said. "Just go to class. I'm not going to report it."

I was grateful for his kindness, but even if he had reported me, I wouldn't have regretted my punch. I couldn't help myself. Everybody knew I was feeling bad already. And truly, I was devastated. I wanted to be a winner so badly, and it just wasn't happening. *Why do I keep losing? Why am I a loser? I'm a loser. I'm always being told I'm not good enough. That guy told me that I can't go to Michigan. This guy told me I cost us the game.*

And then, suddenly, it was like this voice came out of nowhere.

"You took the shot," it said. "The other guys didn't. The whole year, you passed it to Craig. But when it came down to it, you took your shot."

I did, didn't I?

That changed everything for me. EVERYTHING.

From now on, I'm taking my shot, I thought. *No matter what, I'm taking my shot.*

WELL, THE ONLY PROBLEM WAS THAT IN ORDER TO REally take my shot, I had to get out of Flint. My senior year in high school was upon me, and it was time to make my move. Everyone in school knew me as an athlete, but my classmates were always asking me about whatever art project I had in the works, too.

"What's your next painting going to be?" a girl asked me as we walked out of art class together. "Do a Jordan next? Do a Michael Jackson?"

I loved the attention. And I loved art. I wanted to go to the

Center for Creative Studies in Detroit, but there was no way they were going to give me a full-ride art scholarship. Such a thing didn't exist. And they didn't have a football team. So that meant no football scholarship, either. If I went there, I would need to pay my own tuition, and there was no way that was happening.

I had to find a school with a football team that would give me a chance to show everyone what I could do. My small magnet school, Flint Academy, was focused more on academics than athletics, so I had to do anything I could to get even one college to give me a look. I made a big list of possible colleges, and in the end, I wrote to more than a hundred schools in an attempt to gain a scholarship. And this was before I had a computer with a printer, so I wrote them by hand, one at a time.

Before long, letters started coming back to me:

Thank you for your interest in Penn State. We are sorry . . .
Thank you for your interest in USC. We are sorry . . .

They were all rejection letters, except for one. Illinois State actually contacted my high school football coaches and asked to see a tape of me playing. That was a good sign. It was an even better sign when their football coach called me.

"We love you," he said. "We want to give you a scholarship."

I was so excited. I had my Illinois State sweatshirt, and my Illinois State stickers, and I started telling everyone at school all about my future plans.

"I'm going to Illinois State. It's going to be great."

And then it was time for signing day, the day on which the college teams signed all of the high school players they wanted. That day came and went, but my phone never rang. So I called Illinois State and got their football coach on the line.

"Hey, what's going on?" I asked.

"Well, if you'd like to come and walk on, that would be great," he said.

"But I thought . . ."

It turned out there was no scholarship for me. That was so awful. It really hurt. But I knew I had to scramble and try again. My art teacher, Mr. Eichelberg, had been one of the greatest champions of my art talent. He really believed in me as an artist and was as influential for me in art as Coach Lee was when it came to football. He started applying for everything he could on my behalf. We were coming down to the wire when, finally, Western Michigan University came back with a $500 art excellence scholarship.

"Okay, I'll take it," I said. "They want me."

Well, after that, I looked into Western Michigan University's football team and saw they'd had a superstar linebacker, John Offerdahl, who had been drafted by the NFL and was playing for the Miami Dolphins. To me, the fact that he could go pro from there proved that I could do it, too. It wasn't the University of Michigan. It wasn't Michigan State. Those were the two big schools. But I hadn't even been able to gain entry to Michigan State's high school football camp. So I had to be realistic about my options and accept that I was going to have to walk on to the Western Michigan University football team. That was my only way out of Flint.

I went home and told my mother they had given me this little bit of money. It wasn't much, but I hoped it would be enough for me to at least get started.

"You have a year to earn your scholarship," she said.

So that was it, I had one year. By that point, I would have done anything to get out of town, and out of my house. Before my high school graduation, we had an awards ceremony at my high school. My relationship with Big Terry and Trish was so acrimonious by that point that they didn't attend, even though I had invited them. I was voted most likely to succeed, and I was being given the school's highest honor, The Spirit Award. As I heard my name announced, and I strode onto the stage to accept my plaque, all I could think was: *My parents are not here.* Maybe they didn't realize what a big deal it was. Maybe Trish wanted to teach me a lesson. Maybe Big Terry thought I'd gotten too full of myself. That was it. I was more than ready to go.

NOW THAT I'D GRADUATED FROM HIGH SCHOOL, AND I was almost eighteen, Trish couldn't control me anymore. I finally got to go on a date. Throughout my last three years of school, I'd been close friends with three white girls who hung out together, and over the years, I'd had a crush on all of them at one time or another.

During my senior year, I'd been hanging out in the halls with all three when I was called into my high school guidance counselor's office, about a matter of utmost importance. The counselor was a very pretty black woman who was the object of many adolescent daydreams among the boys of Flint Academy.

As I sat in her office, I measured her tone, which was very serious. She sighed.

"Terry, you have a very bright future," she said. "I just want to warn you about one thing I see you doing that could become a big problem for you."

I perked up in a major way. I couldn't wait to hear what this life-altering problem was, and what I could do to fix it.

"Terry—stay away from white women," she continued. "They are no good. They are just going to lead you down a path to destruction."

"Really?" I said, trying to sound respectful.

"Yes. Listen to me. You have no idea how conniving and evil they can be."

Wow. This was the biggest, best advice she thought she could give me about my future. And it was pure nonsense.

"I hear you. Thank you."

I'd avoided her until the school year finally ended.

Now I was out of school. I was a grown man. I called one of the three girls, Sophia. "Would you like to go out with me?" I asked. "You know, why don't we go to a movie and get some pizza?"

"I would love to," she said.

I was totally freaked out because, even though I was seventeen years old and about to leave for college, it was my first date. At least we were already friends and used to hanging out at school together. We laughed and had fun during Rodney Dangerfield's movie *Back to School,* and as we ate pizza, and then we parked in front of Sophia's house. We were listening to Janet Jackson's "Funny How Time Flies (When You're Having Fun)," and I was so happy. Everything was going so well.

"Hey, Sophia, this is cool," I said. "Thank you. I had a great evening."

And then we kissed. It was my first kiss, and I was done. I was in love.

"Bye, Terry," she said as she climbed out of the car.

"Bye, Sophia," I said.

But what I was thinking was: *I would die for you.*

I floated home. There hadn't been any sex, and I was glad. I didn't want any of that to corrupt the way I felt for her. To me, pornography was dirty. And this was pure. She cared. I cared. I didn't want to mess any of that up. Our kiss was perfect.

———

'D RECEIVED A FULL SCHOLARSHIP TO A PRESTIGIOUS SUM-
mer arts program, Interlochen Center for the Arts, located in
northwest Michigan, and I left for six weeks soon after my date.
Interlochen was a seismic shift for me. So many talented, creative people have gone there, from Dermot Mulroney to Mike
Wallace to Norah Jones, and it meant a great deal to me to be in
such illustrious company. Interlochen was also my first immer-
sion in another culture. I was living outside of the city for the
first time. I met people from California and Germany. I also
took my first video production class, in which I made a rap video
with my Flint Academy classmate Ron Croudy, who is still a
close friend to this day. After this experience, I was more convinced than ever that I'd make it to the world of entertainment
someday. On top of that, during a group competition among
ten of us young artists, a judge from the Art Institute of Cincin-
nati picked my drawings as the best. That was a really important affirmation of my artistic talent, and I savored the joy of
receiving his praise. But before I could turn my attention to my
love of arts and entertainment, I had a college football scholarship to win. And before that, I had a girl to see, and maybe kiss
again.

We had no cell phones back then, so I wrote Sophia long
letters all summer. She sent me one letter, and then, just like
that, I didn't receive any more letters from her. I kept writing,
but she didn't write back. When I was able to call her from the
pay phone, she was always busy. But I didn't let that dampen my
feelings, or my hope.

As soon as I got home from Interlochen, the first thing I did
was go to the phone and call Sophia. I was so happy just to hear
her voice.

"Hey, I'm home," I said. "Can we go out? I figured we could do something."

She paused for a long moment.

"I'm sorry. I have a date. We can't go out."

"But I thought—"

"No, Terry, we'd be better off just being friends."

I was crushed. I mean we're talking about the first girl I'd ever kissed, and six weeks of buildup about all of the things we were going to do together, and how I would see her on my school breaks and visit her when she went away to college the following year. I had a whole scenario laid out in my mind, and in my heart. Because I'd never gone through this when I should have, at age thirteen, or sixteen, I was very naive. I was stunted. And then, just like that, my heart was broken.

I didn't realize it at the time, but as I hung up the phone and went back to my room, all of these horrible feelings from my childhood were being stirred up inside of me, feelings that I was worthless and unlovable, feelings that if I wasn't absolutely perfect, then no one would ever love me. All I knew at the time was that I felt unwanted. I hated it. And I never wanted to feel that way again. So I made a vow to myself:

I have to be someone. I have to get out of Flint. I have to make it so somebody will want me. And then I'll show everybody.

Soon after that, my father drove me up to Western Michigan University, and I set it out for him just as clearly as if I were reading directions from the map.

"I'm gonna be a pro football player," I said.

"Well, you know, only one in a million makes it," he said.

"I'm one in a million," I said. "I'm one in a million."

"Okay," he said, not exactly sounding convinced.

"Yep," I said, rolling my eyes at him and his doubts.

I had no use for anyone telling me the odds. I didn't care. I knew I was going to make it because I knew I would do whatever it took. Not only that, but I decided to use any bit of rejection I'd ever received as fuel. Looking back, I'm not sure how healthy that was. But at the time, it worked. It made me work out harder, lift more, and strive to be somebody. And I never, ever stopped, even when it got tough—and let me tell you, it got a lot tougher for a long time before it started to get easier.

WHEN I HIT WESTERN MICHIGAN AND TRIED TO GO right into football camp, the coaches told me I had basically missed it while I'd been at Interlochen. They let me join the team as a walk-on and be a part of the practice squad, but I had to really fight my way up from the bottom. And so I got beat up, literally. But I didn't care. I had my little art scholarship, and my mother was paying for the rest for a year, and I was just so happy to have my pads on.

I knew it was up to me to earn a scholarship to cover the rest of college. From my first practice, I was doing my thing, hitting people. *BOOM. BOOM. BOOM. BOOM.* It was a challenge, but I loved it. Like I said, I never minded hard work when there was a clear purpose and something to be gained.

Football was great, but the rest of my college experience was a major disappointment, almost immediately. After being under my mother's strict control for so many years, I was sure I was going to go crazy as soon as I tasted my first bit of freedom. That lasted for about a week, and my version of wild was tame compared to what we've come to see as the normal college experience. From my first night at school, it seemed like everyone around me was falling-down drunk. I immediately thought of Big Terry and knew I didn't want to be that foolish.

"I'm not drinking," I said.

That was fine. No one was going to force me to drink. But the problem was, all that drinking turned me off from everyone else. I didn't like being around drunk people, and so there really weren't many people for me to be around. But I wanted to be around somebody. So I joined the Western Michigan University branch of the Maranatha Campus Ministries, which was keen on a brand of Christianity called discipleship. Given my extremely religious upbringing, this world felt safe to me. As much as I'd wanted to rebel from Trish, now that I was on my own, I was drawn back into the same strict structure without even being conscious of it. I truly believed in my heart that something horrible would happen to me if I didn't do right by God, and so it felt comfortable to join a church where everyone lived by the same beliefs. It was like the island of misfit toys, a group of people who were hurt and broken, but when we were together it was easier for us than it was in the outside world.

And so, at first, I didn't protest when my new pastor told me I couldn't listen to the rap music I loved. And when I was instructed that, if there was a girl I wanted to date, I should go through our pastor to make sure God wanted us to be together, I opted not to date. As long as I had a few people to hang out with on the weekends, I was fine. My main obsession was earning a place on the football team, and from there, a scholarship, and I didn't want anything else to distract me.

I was working extremely hard and putting a tremendous amount of pressure on myself, and so when I felt overly stressed, I began acting out in familiar ways. When my roommate left for the weekend, I snuck out to the drugstore and bought porn. And then, before he came back to school, I put it in the trash. I felt really guilty and threw myself more resolutely into the church, but my prayers never made me stop. I didn't share my problem with anyone, and so I just learned to live with it.

———

DID VERY WELL DURING THE FALL FOOTBALL SEASON, BUT then the university had a coaching change, and I had to win over a whole new crop of coaches. That spring, we had a second football camp, and this was a major moment for me. I had to earn my scholarship in order to come back in the fall. If I didn't, that was the end of college for me. I threw myself into that camp. I was outrunning, outjumping, outlifting all of the other guys. I played my heart out. I mean I really did everything I could.

Finally, my linebacker coach had had enough.

"Somebody beat Terry Crews," he screamed at the other players.

He wanted to prove I wasn't good enough for a scholarship, but I didn't care. People were trying so hard to beat me. They were throwing up all around me. They were passing out. But I just worked that much harder. I wasn't going to let anybody beat me. I knew this was my way out. And I actually impressed the coaches. This was the beginning of me seeing how fitness could help me determine my own destiny. Not only could it change my body, but it could also change the way people viewed me and what I could do. And so it could change the opportunities I had in my life.

I had high hopes when I met with Coach. I sat down across from him and looked at him expectantly. We talked for a little while, and then I came right out and asked him for an athletic scholarship. He broke it down for me.

"You're not good enough," he said. "If you want to stay, it will have to be on your own dime. And if you want to leave, well, good luck."

I was hurt and disappointed. My parents couldn't afford to pay for another year of school. I'd promised to earn a scholarship, and I'd failed. That summer, I returned to the harsh reality of life in Flint. The once-booming auto factories that had been the lifeblood of the city's economy were continuing to be phased out one by one. Crack was the drug of choice for users and dealers. If I didn't find a way out, soon, I'd be trapped. I heard Coach Lee's voice in my head, and I knew I couldn't give up. Football, for me, was never the end goal. It was always a means. Without it, I had no way to go anywhere. I begged my parents, particularly my mother, to give me one more chance, one more semester to try and earn a full-ride scholarship.

Trish was in the kitchen washing dishes. She threw down her dish towel.

"Why do you have to dream so large?" she asked. "I can't stand to see you be so disappointed all of the time, to always be wanting more and never get it."

I stared back at her, feeling guilty. I knew it seemed unfair to ask them to focus so much money and attention on what I was trying to do, when Marcelle and Micki had needs, too. But I don't think I really understood at the time exactly how much of a strain I was putting on my parents. All I knew was that, if I succeeded, not only would my tuition be paid for, but I would also be truly independent of them.

"Please," I said.

"You know, Terry, I'm just going to give you one more semester," she said. "That's all I can afford. Right now, we're already in debt, and it's bad. I can't hold this burden anymore. I really can't hold it."

That was a heavy thing to take on, but I was so relieved.

"I'm gonna make it," I said. "You'll see."

THAT SUMMER, MY FATHER SAID I NEEDED TO GET A JOB. I told him I wanted to be in movies and TV. The only thing resembling that in Flint at the time was the local ABC affiliate, WJRT-TV12. So Big Terry took me down to the station with some of my drawings and paraded me in front of the receptionist.

"My son's an artist," he said. "He'd like to get a job here."

"O-kay . . . let me get someone who can help you," she said, keeping a wary eye on us both. I just wanted to get through this embarrassment. I was sure we were about to get kicked out of there.

The visual arts director came out and Big Terry said the exact same thing. One of Big Terry's best traits is his consistency. The director looked at my portfolio.

"When can he start?" he asked.

I couldn't believe it. I worked at Channel 12 all summer, drawing backdrops for newscasts and coming up with ideas for anything that required creativity. I even cleaned up around the station when it needed it. Then I got my big break, replacing their usual courtroom-sketch guy during the biggest murder case in Flint at the time. The station manager loved my work and told me if I ever needed any help in this business, to give him a call. My first job in entertainment was a success.

N AUGUST OF 1987, I PUT MY CLOTHES IN GARBAGE BAGS and headed back to Western Michigan University for football camp. The pressure was on. Hustling hard in practice, I would not be ignored. Still undersized and skinny, I worked out in the dormitory weight room on my own and was inspired by the athletes who walked around campus in the letterman's jackets distributed by the athletic department.

I earned the right to play in games that year and was the only walk-on player to do so. After a five-win, six-loss record, and with one week left in the semester, I waited for my scholarship offer but heard nothing. Finally, I needed to know where my future stood, so I scheduled a meeting with the head coach.

I entered his office and sat across from him at his enormous desk. He looked up as if he had better things to do. I plowed ahead.

"Coach, my parents can't afford to pay for school anymore," I said. "If I'm going to continue playing for the university, it will have to be on scholarship."

"We don't have any more scholarships left," he said.

I could barely make out his words as he said something about "getting on financial aid." I nodded but couldn't speak.

"I'm sorry, there's nothing else I can do," he said.

"Thank you," I said, already standing.

I got on my bike and rode back to my dorm room. I'd made a promise to my family, and I'd blown it. I'd asked my parents to gamble, and I'd wasted all of their money, which they couldn't afford to lose. *Maybe I can go to art school,* I thought. I knew asking my parents to sacrifice again was out of the question. I had no choice but to go home and work. But all of the factories were closed. And even though Channel 12 might be a possibility, I didn't want anything to tie me down to Flint. If I was going to be broke, I at least wanted to be broke in a place I could love.

I was flailing. I didn't know what I was going to do. Finally, there was no putting it off any longer. I gathered up my clothes and put them into garbage bags. I tied them up and stacked them against the wall. I called my parents to tell them the disappointing news and made arrangements for them to pick me up after my last exam. My college dream was over, and with it my football dream, too.

2

JUST KEEP GOING

WORK

CHAPTER 6

NO IS NEGOTIABLE

HAD PUSHED MYSELF SO HARD. I HAD AIMED TO BE perfect. And I had failed. I hadn't earned a scholarship, and my time in college was over. With the threat of my return to Flint looming, and the fear of my empty future pressing down on me, I wanted something, anything, to make the pressure go away.

I thought of the campus ministry I belonged to and the pledge I'd made to give myself over to God. That was what I needed to do, devote myself with even greater dedication to my beliefs and my community. I was in my Zimmerman Hall dormitory room, feeling restless and low-down, when I noticed a girl go into the room next door. We talked occasionally when we bumped into each other around the dorm. I took a deep breath, put on a smile I didn't really feel, and walked over to her open doorway. "Hey, what's up?" I said.

"Hey, Terry," she said, smiling back at me.

"You busy?" I said.

She invited me in, and we both sat down on beanbags near the room's wooden, loft-style configuration. Her roommate had already left for winter break. We made small talk as usual, but then I started talking about my life, and how I didn't know what I was going to do next. We were listening to Michael Jackson's "The Lady in My Life," and as time stretched on, it was clear that neither one of us wanted to go. The next thing I knew, we were kissing, and then we were both stretched out on the carpet. Even as it was happening, I knew it was wrong, but I didn't stop. For one perfect moment, my mind achieved that blankness I craved, the one I got from pornography. And then neither of us had any clothes on, and suddenly, I was very aware of being there with her. I knew I shouldn't be doing this. There were many moments I could have stopped. Many moments I should have. But I felt like this was my chance to see what sex was all about. Finally, I was touching a real woman. We kept going and going until, eventually, I just stopped.

"Is that it?" I asked, the question more to myself than to her.

"Are you done?" she said.

"I don't know, I didn't . . ." I said.

I didn't know anything, really. I was more confused than ever, and now the guilt was sinking in. I wanted to get away from her, away from the place where I'd gone against everything I'd been taught, and everything I'd believed in, and away from myself. I pulled on my clothes as quickly as I could, hardly looking at her as I ducked out of her room. *How did that happen? How did that happen? How did that happen?* The question kept working its way through my mind with no answer, and no resolution, and no end to my torment as I hurried into the shower and stood there under the hot water.

For so long, I'd been waiting to have sex, and fantasizing

about sex, and thinking about the kind of woman I wanted to marry and have sex with, and now it had finally happened, but it hadn't been at all like I'd wanted it to be. I was so disappointed. *Is that it?* I wondered again.

I felt contempt for the girl I'd slept with, but of course, even as immature and inexperienced as I was back then, I knew the person I really despised was myself.

And the worst part was that my circumstances were just as hopeless as they'd been before I went into her room. At the end of the week, I had to go back to Flint, for good, and I couldn't stand the thought. Everything collapsed. I was beyond hoping that things would be better once I got home. I was beyond everything.

On Thursday, I was in my dorm room when I was called to the phone at the end of the hall. I figured it was my pastor or someone from home. I didn't think I could bear to talk to any of them, not with the shame of what I'd done coloring everything, but I forced myself to pick up the receiver and see who was on the line. I was surprised when I was greeted by a deep voice. It was the head coach.

"Terry, we want you to come by the office," he said. "I've got to talk to you."

"Sure, I'll be right over," I said.

The coach's office was the last place I wanted to go, as it was just one more reminder of my defeat, but as I pulled on my coat, I couldn't help but wonder what his call could mean. Maybe they'd found me a partial scholarship. I knew it was dangerous to hope, though, as I doubted anything less than a full ride would be enough for Trish to let me stay. The walkways were too icy for me to ride my bike, and the winter air was frigid. I hunched my shoulders and hustled over to the athletics building. When I sat down across from the coach, he looked at me sternly. It felt like my humiliation would never end. I just hoped he'd get it over with quickly.

"Terry, we found one more scholarship," he said. "One more."

I don't remember the next part of our conversation. It was like I was suddenly having an out-of-body experience. Finally, I pulled myself together.

"I'm on scholarship," I said, still in shock.

"Yes, we have a scholarship for you."

"Can I see it?"

I almost couldn't believe it was true until I saw the words in writing.

"Yeah, we have all the paperwork," he said. "We want you to go see the secretary and sign."

"Thank you," I said, standing and shaking his hand.

The coach was barely smiling at me, acting instead like he was some kind of magnanimous benefactor, reluctantly granting my request for a scholarship, but I knew he would never regret his decision. I had earned my place on the team, and now I would earn my scholarship, by playing harder and with more heart than I'd ever played before.

As I hurried back across the blustery campus, I could hardly feel the cold weather anymore. I couldn't wait to call my parents and tell them I'd made good on my promise after all. Nearing my dorm, I thought of the substitute teacher in high school who'd never believed I could make it. I'd proved him wrong. And then I thought of Coach Lee, the first one to believe in me and plant the seed of my dream. I had done it. I had earned a full-ride scholarship at a Division One university. I had sweated, and fought, and in the end, the coaches hadn't been willing to lose me.

As soon as I reached my dorm, I went right to the phone.

"Ma, I did it," I said. "You don't have to pay for college anymore. My college is paid for."

Being able to tell my mother she had been right to believe in me was the best feeling in the world. I still get emotional when I think about that phone call today, more than twenty-five years later. Thanks to that one moment in my life, everything changed. The way I'd grown up in Flint, you either had it or you didn't. You were either good at math or you sucked. You were either a foreman or you were on the line. There was no mingling between the two, and there was no chance to work your way over to the other side. In fact, if you tried for more, everybody would put you in your place as fast as they could, like, "Who do you think you are? You think you're gonna do that? They're not gonna let you."

But at that moment right after I earned my scholarship, I stopped and thought: *Wait a minute. No is negotiable. I can actually change where I go and how I get there. I can actually make my way over to the other side. It's up to me.* And all I did was I didn't quit. Even when it was over, I kept looking for another way. If I'd listened to the negative answers people kept giving me, that would have been it. If I'd been depressed and given up when my scholarship didn't happen the previous fall, that would have been it. But I took it to the end. And finally, a door opened.

That was a huge epiphany for me. I was hooked on the possibility of having that kind of next-level experience again and again. My one victory made me want bigger and better, and suddenly, the whole world opened up with possibility for me.

I can just keep doing this, I thought. *Now, if I just keep going, nobody can stop me. Even if someone tells me I can't do something in the future, I'm not going to listen. I'm just going to keep on moving. And that way, I'll be unstoppable.*

What had been the end of higher education for me was now

just Christmas vacation. I went home, and we celebrated the biggest victory of my life so far.

THE GOOD FEELINGS DIDN'T LAST LONG. I RETURNED TO school that January, prepared to work harder than I'd ever worked in my life. As I said, I've never shied away from extreme exertion, as long as it's for a purpose, so that didn't put me off at all. What I wasn't prepared for were back-to-back experiences of disillusionment in the two areas of my life that had gotten me this far: football and faith.

As much time as I'd spent dreaming about my football scholarship, I'd been totally ignorant as to what the reality would be like. And my return to school was a rude awakening. First of all, I hadn't realized that a college scholarship is a full-time job. More than full-time, it's twenty-four hours a day. We weren't allowed to seek out any other form of employment during the school year, so I was totally dependent on the football team for all I had. My coaches became my father, my mother, my everything. This was not a comfortable situation for a nineteen-year-old college sophomore, especially one with problems accepting responsibility. Here I had asked for, worked for, and finally received this scholarship, but instead of feeling grateful, I quickly acquired a sense of entitlement. Even worse, with how much I was practicing and working out, even before the football season started, I wasn't concentrating on my schoolwork. Football had become my entire life, and I was so full of my sense of entitlement that I became resentful of the classes I needed to take in order to play. I began to feel the school should take care of me. I became angry—hostile even—toward the very people who had given me an opportunity. My bad attitude began to rub people the wrong way, and then I started to feel like the coaches had it in for me. I went back and forth between being grateful that I wasn't stuck in Flint and bristling at the restrictions put on my life by my coaches.

The problems with my church life weren't easy to accept, either. Feeling confused and guilty, I'd gone to my pastor after I lost my virginity. If I'd been a little put off by the way he pressed me for the intimate details of what had gone down, I was so focused on blaming myself for my misdeeds that I was mostly just glad to have someone to pray with and help me get back on the right path.

And then I went to Dallas with my pastor and the others in our church for a big conference of all the campus ministries. The centerpiece of the event featured a black pastor who introduced the guests of honor, who were essentially the mother and father of our church, and who also happened to be white. Amid applause from the audience, the church mother took the podium and spoke.

"We have to thank God," she said. "We have to be grateful for the love of God, and for Christianity, and for all of you being saved, because if it weren't for Christianity, all of you would be worshipping idols in the jungle."

The members of the college ministries who were in attendance were predominantly African American, and it was as if there was a single collective snap in the audience, followed by the thought: *She did not just say that.*

I couldn't believe it. As I tried to process what she'd just revealed about the church I'd devoted myself to, I didn't hear another word she spoke. After she was done speaking, the black pastor returned to the stage.

"Now, you all know we needed to hear that," he said.

No, I thought. *The Kool-Aid may have gotten to you, but not to me.*

Everything was different from that moment forward. I didn't know what I was going to do yet, but I knew something had to change in a major way. I went back to the hotel where we were all staying, and someone from our ministry told me that my pastor wanted to talk to me down in one of the conference rooms. I walked into the room, expecting to see my pastor seated at the conference table waiting for me. Instead, ten pastors, including my pastor, sat in chairs in a semicircle, while one single chair sat empty across from them, as if it was some kind of tribunal.

Instantly uncomfortable, I stood awkwardly behind the chair.

One of the pastors gave me a hard look.

"We heard about your infidelity," he said.

I looked at my pastor. "What?" I asked, incredulous.

"I told them about what you did," he said. "And now we're going to get over this together. These men are going to help you to overcome your demons."

"Okay," I said, feeling uneasy, but sitting in the chair, as they'd indicated.

"Terry, you know that's wrong, right?" another pastor said. "Sexual sin is something that will take you out for the rest of your life."

One at a time, they all lit into me, telling me I'd done wrong.

"You were representing this church," another pastor said. "You are one of our leaders, and you cannot behave in this way."

I already knew what I'd done didn't line up with my beliefs and the person I wanted to be. I felt bad enough as it was. And now I'd been betrayed. I pretended to listen, but I was already gone. Finally, I couldn't take it anymore. I looked over at my pastor. *You're the guy who said don't tell a lie,* I thought. *Let's start*

*with that. You said you wouldn't tell anybody, and you told ten peo-
ple, at least.*

My pastor caught my expression.

"You needed it," he said, giving me the smuggest look.

After what the church mother had said, and now this, I felt
empty. My pastor was my ride back to school, so I kept my
mouth shut. I went to the rest of the events. I endured the drive
home. I played nice, shook hands, and acted all kumbaya.

But as soon as I got back to my dorm room and closed the
door behind me, it was a wrap. When I didn't show up for the
next meeting, I started getting phone calls from my pastor and
the other members of our church. I didn't go to the next meeting, either, and my phone wouldn't stop ringing. Finally, I answered.

"I'm gone," I said. "It's not working."

"Well, you know, Terry, you're making the wrong move," he
said. "God's not going to let you go."

He proceeded to tell me all of the scary stuff that was going
to happen to me if I left the church. But I was tired of being
threatened by people I didn't respect.

"Well, it's just gonna have to happen, because I'm not coming back," I said.

"I'm sorry, man."

Instead of feeling elated that I'd stood up for myself, I was
devastated. I was the loneliest I've ever been. Because I'd joined
a church group that looked down on our classmates as sinners,
I'd never made any friends. I didn't hang out with the football
team. I was completely alone.

———

L UCKILY, I DID HAVE ONE FRIEND, JOSEPH APPLEWHITE, who lived near me in the Zimmerman Hall dormitory. He was at Western Michigan on a track scholarship for the long jump, and this brother could leap and fly like a gazelle, yet he never really cared about his athletic ability. He was as laid back as I was driven. When he first got to school, he'd visited a Maranatha meeting and decided it wasn't for him, and so he understood what Maranatha was all about. He was the only person I felt like I could talk with about what had happened, and his perspective was a lifeline for me. Not long after my phone call with my pastor, I started worrying that I'd made the wrong decision. Even though I knew I couldn't associate with people I didn't fundamentally agree with, it was even harder not to associate with anyone. I needed a deprogramming, and without it, I was afraid the bad things my pastor had predicted would happen. I was bereft. I was scared. For the first few weeks, I was a zombie.

Finally, Joe invited me to go with him and his girlfriend, April, to another area church, the Christian Life Center, for their Wednesday night service. Even though I felt like a third wheel, I was so lonely I would have accepted any invitation.

We arrived at a very small, traditional-looking white church on Kalamazoo's north side. As we entered amid the requisite churchlike smell of Pine-Sol, I noticed three women we'd think of now as Real Housewives of Kalamazoo singing into wireless mics. The music was really good, not religious-sounding at all, with a definite groove that made me nod my head. Then I saw the pianist. She was bowed over the keys of a late-model synthesizer like Schroeder from *Peanuts.* Only she was really pretty. She was skinny, with very short, curly hair, and as she glanced up to connect with the singers, I strained to guess her ethnicity. Her hair was sandy brown, with scattered blond highlights, and she had high cheekbones and a slight overbite that made her look very exotic. With her olive skin, I suspected she was Hispanic. Whatever she was, she was beautiful. She left the keyboard and sat a few rows ahead of me.

It felt good to be there, away from the dormitory and all of its raucous, juvenile behavior, in a place that felt clean, like everyone in the room was trying to be a better person. As the pastor spoke, I stole looks at the keyboard player.

"Amen," she said, leaning forward. "Amen."

Maybe she was the pastor's keyboard-playing, sermon-agreeing wife. Feeling guilty, I averted my eyes. But I couldn't keep them away for long.

When I made a move to leave at the evening's end, Joe held me back.

"There's someone I want you to meet," he said.

I nodded absently, my eyes instantly returning to the keyboard player. Just then, someone handed her a little blond baby. Now I was really in trouble. She was someone's wife, someone's mother. I tried to distract myself by looking for whoever Joe wanted me to meet. That's when Joe waved over the woman I'd been admiring.

"This is my friend, Terry," he said. "Terry, this is Rebecca."

Her soft, brown eyes seemed to disappear into her smile. With her small baby planted firmly on her hip, it was as if she and the little girl were one. She extended her free hand to me, and I shook it in the most respectful way possible.

"Wow, you can really play that keyboard."

"Oh, thank you," she said. "Thank you."

Okay, so I wasn't exactly pulling off anything in the vicinity of suave, but she was really pretty. I did my best to make conversation until she turned to talk to Joe. As they spoke, I was too busy looking at Rebecca to really follow their conversation. I wondered how this mysterious woman with the little blond baby had ended up in this predominantly African-American congregation, and why I couldn't stop looking at her, even though she didn't seem the least bit interested in me.

When we got out to the car, I grilled Joe for information. He told me that Rebecca wasn't with her daughter's father and was a single mom.

Okay, I don't feel so bad, now that I know she's single, I thought. *That's a start.*

Not that I had any idea what it might be a start of, as I was a nineteen-year-old college student who'd never had a girl-friend and was hopeless around the house: I couldn't even fry an egg.

Joe and April often came and knocked on my dorm room door because Joe knew I was lonely. We would always roll to this burger place, Elias Brothers Big Boy. The next time we went, Rebecca was there, too. I was glad to see her, and not only because she was pretty, but also because talking to her made me feel less like I was Joe and April's charity case. This time, Rebecca and I had the best time together, just laughing and talking about life, and school, and everything. I was starting to really like her, but then I'd look at her and remember: *You've got a baby. There's no way I'm ready for that. I don't know anything about anything.*

For the next few months, it seemed like Joe was always inviting me out to places where we happened to run into Rebecca. Of course I later found out that Joe was trying to hook us up. But at the time, Rebecca and I were just enjoying the experience of getting to know each other.

Meanwhile, I began to attend the Christian Life Center

church. As much as I liked everyone there, after what I'd been through with Maranatha, I had decided I would never again give myself over completely to any organization. I would always keep something back for myself. Of course, no one at my new church had any interest in controlling me, and I was glad to have finally found a real community.

I stayed in Kalamazoo that summer to work at a refrigeration company, Stafford-Smith, owned by one of my teammate's fathers. I moved in with another Maranatha defector, Mike Lewis, who had a beautiful apartment on Lovell Street.

There was an additional benefit to my new church. They frequently held picnics and singles events, and when I showed up, Rebecca was always there. One night, we all went bowling. I looked over and saw Rebecca at the top of one of the lanes, and I noticed she had really nice legs. *Whoo-whee, look at those legs,* I thought. But always, any admiring thought was followed by a reality check: *She has a baby.*

As I got to know Rebecca better, and learned more about her situation, both my sympathy and admiration for her increased. The former Miss Gary 1984, she'd been a musical theater major with a 4.0 grade point average when she became pregnant. She hadn't been dating her baby's father, and she considered giving her baby up for adoption, but she couldn't do it. When it became clear the father was incapable of helping her to raise her daughter, she dropped out of college and went on welfare while she completed beauty school.

Even though she was determined, and she worked incredibly hard, she was really struggling, and she'd gotten in the habit of calling Joe when she needed help with something. So now both Joe and I went to her aid. She had this old beater car that was always breaking down, and so Joe and I often showed up and pushed it for her. One time, we called her a tow truck.

When it came, the driver hooked up her car incorrectly, and it wrecked her car. The poor woman could not get a break.

"Oh, whatever, it doesn't matter," she said.

It mattered to me. I chewed out the tow truck guy. I just felt so much for her and her situation. As Joe and I were leaving her house that day, I turned to him.

"When I go pro, I'm going to buy that girl a car," I said.

"Really?" he said.

"Yep, when I go pro, I'm going to buy her a car. I hope her husband doesn't get mad at me."

I honestly thought she'd be married to someone else by that point, because she was two years older than me, and I knew getting married and raising a kid was way more than I was capable of then. But she was beautiful, and she didn't have a man, and she'd had to call the cops on her daughter's father before, and knowing all of this, and how much I liked her, I really wanted to see her make it.

I may have been altruistic when it came to Rebecca, but not so much regarding my family. Along with my new sense of accomplishment after I earned my scholarship, I'm not proud to admit that I also felt like I deserved special treatment within my family. I was never above begging and pleading for what I wanted until Trish and Big Terry couldn't stand it anymore and finally gave in to my demands.

Now that I'd made good on my promise to them and earned my scholarship, I was sure I was on my way to the NFL, and my attitude was that I was the guy in our family who was going to become a star and achieve greatness for all of us. And because of this, I decided I needed a car, and they needed to buy it for me. Trish had not been exaggerating about the amount of debt they'd accrued keeping me in college, and she wasn't in a position to give me anything right then, no matter how much of a pain I was about it. So I went to my grandmother. "I went and got a scholarship, and now I need you to help me get a car," I said.

"Uh, well, how are you gonna pay me for this?" she asked.

"We're going to get money for the scholarship, and I'll pay you back," I said.

Maybe I really did have the intention of working during the summer and making good on my promise, but I honestly would have said anything to get what I wanted. The reality is you get zero points for intentions. You only get points for behavior, and I was behaving like a petulant child. I believe Mama knew her money wasn't coming back, but she gave in to my demands anyhow because I was so good at convincing others to give me what I needed. I used my scholarship to convince everyone I was going pro. In a sense I was selling my family tickets to my dream. My grandmother agreed to put the down payment on a car for me, and then I was supposed to pay the note on it. I wanted a Jeep, and I'd been telling Rebecca for months that I was going to come back to school with one. But my family at least put practicality before my grandiose view of myself, and they bought me this little Chevy Nova instead. I didn't care, really. I was just so happy to go back to school with a car of my own. It really came in handy for helping out Rebecca and her daughter, Naomi. And with that car came freedom.

But, of course, I ended up not giving anyone in my family a single cent for the note on that car. When they came to me for the money not long after that, I was straight with them. "I don't have it," I said.

And so my mother and father had to take on the whole loan themselves. I didn't think twice about it. I was so sure I was headed for greatness it was almost like I felt they were lucky for being able to help me. Ah, the arrogance of youth. Don't worry. I was about to get brought back down to size, many, many times.

CHAPTER 7

AS SOON AS I GO PRO

'D BEEN WORKING HARD ALL SUMMER, AND THE TASTE of Kalamazoo was coming up. It struck me that I should ask Rebecca if she wanted to go with me. I was lonely. I felt like her days were really dark, considering all she was struggling with, and I was going through some dark days, too. I saw us as really good friends more than anything else at that point. I just wanted to give her some brightness.

She agreed to go out with me. I was so happy and all about getting it right. When I came home from work the night of our date, I got cleaned up, and I carefully laid out my best outfit. I had this awful baggy pink shirt that billowed way out in the back, but I stuffed it into my pants, and I put on this gray tie I had to go with it. At the time, I had a high-top fade with a blond streak, and I made sure that was looking good, too. You know, it was back in the day, and I was all about the hip-hop look.

Mike Lewis saw me getting ready in the bathroom of our apartment.

"You know what?" he said. "I see you and Rebecca together, man."

"Aw, no, man, she's got a baby," I said. "I don't know. I don't see that."

I wasn't going to marry Rebecca, but I was excited to go out with her. As I pulled up in front of her apartment, the sun was shining its golden light down on everything, and it was this beautiful, perfect summer evening. When Rebecca came to the door, I stopped short. She'd done her hair up, and she had on full makeup. I had never seen her like that, and she was gorgeous, I mean stunning.

"What?" she said. "What?"

I was struck dumb.

"Oh, I know this little boy ain't making me blush," she said.

"You look amazing," I said.

"Okay, that's cool," she said.

"Where's Naomi?" I asked.

"With my friend," she said. "You ready?"

I was more than ready. I walked her out to my Chevy Nova, and we headed to downtown Kalamazoo. And then our evening came to an abrupt halt. It was a twenty-one-and-over event. Rebecca was twenty-one. I was only nineteen.

I felt my mood deflate, but Rebecca went right up to the guy at the entrance.

"He's not going to drink," she said. "He doesn't drink."

I perked up and tried to look as innocent as possible.

"I don't drink at all," I said. "I'm with her."

He gave me the up and down. I must have looked desperate. He smiled.

"Aw, go on in."

I was so relieved and grateful. Rebecca moved into the crowd ahead of me.

"Hold on, hold on, let me lead you," I said.

I grabbed her hand and pushed my way through the throng of people, clearing a path for us as I went. Rebecca later told me that this was the moment she felt something between us. I felt it, too, along with the desire to take care of her.

I led her over to an open space where we could dance.

Don't mess it up, I thought. *Don't mess it up.*

I was so respectful of her. I almost didn't want to touch her, even though she was the most beautiful woman I'd ever seen. For me, sex had a dark side because of my secret pornography habit, and because of what had happened with the girl in my dormitory, and how dirty I'd felt afterward. I didn't want any of that to soil what was so good about that moment and how amazing it felt to be with Rebecca. And so I didn't even want to think of her in that way. As we danced, I held her at a distance, just to be safe. *This is somebody's mom,* I thought. *This is a real woman, with a child. And look at her: She's gorgeous. You're out with the real deal. Do not mess it up.*

"Um, you know, you can get closer," she said, smiling at me.

"Really?" I said. "Is it okay?"

"Come on in, it's okay," she said.

I came on in and just sort of laid my chest against her body. The ground went out from under me, the sky lifted up from above me, and I was floating. To this day, I remember everything so clearly, how she felt, and how good she smelled.

Oh my God, I'm actually holding a real woman, and talking with her, and laughing with her, and having a good time, I thought. *This is so beautiful.*

It was the perfect evening. We went for dinner at Great Lakes Shipping Company. I had my cash all ready. I didn't want her to order something nice, and then not have enough money to cover it. *There will be no mistakes,* I thought.

"I've got a nice chunk ready for whatever you want," I said. "You can get whatever you want on the menu."

I guess I don't have to keep telling you how young I was, right?

Rebecca smiled at me and ordered. And then we sat there and talked and talked, and there wasn't one single thing she said that gave me the slightest pause. I looked into her eyes, and I thought: *This is gorgeous. This is bliss.*

I took her home, and I led her into her house. Right before I turned to leave, I was moved to speak.

"You know, Rebecca," I said, "I don't know what this is, or where this is going, but I just want you to know that I'm willing. I don't know, but I'm willing."

"Okay," she said. "Okay."

Before that night, all I'd been able to see were obstacles: *I'm too young. You're too much of a mom. You've got a baby. I can't do any of that.* But by the end of our first date, I had no apprehensions at all. I knew everything would take care of itself.

When I got home, my roommate, Mike, was still up.

"How'd it go?" he asked.

"Man, it's all good," I said. "You know, it went great. It was good."

"I see you two," he said again.

"No, no, no, don't go there," I said. "Look, man, I'm trying to tell you, I don't know what's going to happen. She may not like me. She may turn around and whatever, I don't know. But it was a great night."

I knew I could mess everything up by trying to analyze the situation too much, and I just wanted to enjoy the moment for what it was while it lasted.

W E WERE SOON INSEPARABLE: REBECCA AND ME. AND Naomi. It was a big life lesson for me, for sure. We spent hours over at Rebecca's house, with Naomi sitting in her little seat, as cute as could be. But when she got grumpy, I had to learn to be patient. When Rebecca was at her house, and I was at mine, we talked on the phone, and I mean late into the night. It was one of those scenarios where we stayed on the phone until we were both falling asleep. She had the best voice ever, the sexiest, most beautiful voice. I was in love with that voice. But I hadn't yet gotten clear on my feelings about Rebecca. I'd just turned twenty years old, and I'd never been allowed to date, so I was stunted in the extreme. This was my first girlfriend, and it took me a little while to catch up with her. Finally, after several months, Rebecca got real with me one day while we were talking on the phone.

"What are you feeling?" she said. "What do you feel about me?"

Now, my whole life I'd been told that I couldn't date, but I'd eventually find a woman to marry and have a family with, and when I'd been in Maranatha, they'd told me if I wanted to even just date a woman, I had to get clearance from my pastor in order to be sure God really wanted us to be together. So that's how I thought.

"Please don't get offended," I said. "But I think you're supposed to be my wife. I just, I really do."

"Really?" she said.

"I do," I said. "I don't know what's happening. But I know I feel like we were always meant to be together. I don't know how to be a father. I don't know how to be a husband. I don't know any of this. But I'm willing. You make me want to do things I never thought I could do."

"Wow," she said.

I went over to her place that night, and as soon as I walked in, we kissed. And then she pulled back and looked at me.

"You know what?" she said. "I'm with that, too. I want us to be together."

That right there was our engagement. The next time we saw our pastor I couldn't help but beam at him.

"We're engaged," I said.

"That's kind of quick," he said. "I mean, you guys hung out for six months."

"I know," I said.

Rebecca's mother flipped.

"What?" Rebecca's mother said to her. "You're getting married to this boy? He doesn't have anything. What are you doing?"

My mother flipped. She had been in the same situation as Rebecca, a single mom, who wasn't quite making it on her own. And she was afraid, as she'd always been, that a woman looking for a daddy for her baby would trap me. But I wasn't going to let anyone tell me what to feel or how to live. I'd made up my mind.

"I love her," I said. "And I know this is the decision I'm ready to make. I'm going to be with her, and we're going to do this together, forever."

Over the summer, I took Rebecca to Flint to meet my parents and my grandmother, and they treated her so coldly. At first, they did not like her at all. Rebecca is very independent, and she does not care what other people think of her, and that was in direct opposition to how my mother lived and expected

Rebecca and everyone else to behave. One day, Rebecca decided she needed a little bit of a tan, so she went out onto the front lawn of my parents' house in a bathing suit. My father went crazy. He ran outside and started yelling and waving his arms.

"Rebecca, get off the front lawn," Big Terry said. "Yo, you are about to get attacked, and I can't help you when these brothers come running over here."

"What?" she said. "I just want to get a tan."

"No, no, get in the house," he said. "You cannot do that here in Flint, Michigan."

She's from Gary, Indiana, which was basically the same kind of city, so she knew she'd be fine, but with him flipping out like that, she ended up going inside.

From the beginning, it was a real clash between everybody. But I actually kind of enjoyed the conflict. For me, it was my stand. It was my declaration of independence. And, of course, that made the situation grate on my mother's nerves even more. But then, slowly but surely, Rebecca sat down and really talked with the women in my family, and they ended up loving her more than they loved me. Really.

Now, the fact that my family had come to love Rebecca and had gotten behind our marriage did not mean I was actually ready to get married. I was naive on so many levels. I didn't know how to save, and I was very bad with money. Rebecca later told me that she saw warning signs from the beginning, but she ignored them because she was swept up in the bliss of dating. Although I worked all summer, I always took my check and spent it on Rebecca, or I went right out and bought new tennis shoes and T-shirts, leaving nothing behind for the bills.

"Yeah, but did you pay your rent?" Rebecca asked me.

"Oh, no, that's going to be taken care of," I said.

That didn't exactly sound like a good plan to her, but she let it be. I don't know who I thought was going to be taking care of my rent, because I certainly wasn't paying it. My best friend, Darwin, had transferred to Western Michigan University and taken over Mike's room in our apartment. I ended up being short on the rent several months in a row, and we had to sneak out in the middle of the night. I still feel horrible about that to this day. Back then I didn't take responsibility for myself or my actions. I thought ignoring a situation was the same as fixing it. Once again, I had such a sense of entitlement that I thought what was good for me was also good for everyone else.

That fall I returned to school as a junior and threw myself into my first season of playing football since I'd earned my scholarship. Coming out of football camp the previous spring, what had once been the greatest thing ever had become something I hated. Now that I knew my scholarship was revocable if I didn't do everything my coaches said, the pressure to conform felt like a heavy burden. It was wild to have gotten what I wanted, and then to despise it so quickly. My mind-set was much like it had been when I lost my virginity. I'd looked at my classmate like she'd used me because I couldn't handle taking responsibility for my own actions. Now I did the same thing with my college coaches, projecting my guilt onto them about the fact that I wasn't handling myself well at all, and becoming angry toward them for what I saw as their controlling and condescending attitude toward me.

This happened around the time I was dating Rebecca, so they understandably began to feel that our relationship was taking me off track. My grades were poor, but I knew that had nothing to do with Rebecca. I'd decided my major would be football and forget the rest. Finally, the coaches called me into their office. "We think you're changing your attitude with that girlfriend of yours," Coach said.

"That is way out of bounds for you to say to any grown man," I said.

"Well, you're having these problems, and we think it's that girlfriend."

"Dude, I don't talk about your wife," I said. "Don't bring my girlfriend's name up in your mouth one more time."

The coaches and I clashed hard from that moment on, and for the rest of my time on the team, it was a nasty conflict. They considered me a rebel and an ingrate, which was the stone-cold truth. I threw all of my resentment and anger into working out and playing harder than ever, and there was no stopping me. I've always said it takes a lot of pain to be a great football player, because your anger can take you a long way on the football field. A guy with two great parents is not very common in the NCAA or NFL. Thousands of young men fuel their athletic careers with the pain of childhood trauma or other rejections, when it should be fueled by inspiration and love of the game. And the problem is, when you're off the field, you're still angry.

I started making a name for myself at our school and beyond, and it became known that the NFL scouts had taken notice. Our team went all the way that season and ended up winning the Mid-American Conference (MAC) championship for 1988. It was our school's first championship in nearly thirty years. I was really starting to feel like my entrance to the NFL was on the verge of happening, and so I did my best to stay positive.

My future looked bright, but my present circumstances were not. Without a place of my own, I moved in with Rebecca. She had a government-subsidized apartment because she was a single mom, and I wasn't really supposed to be there, so I snuck in and out. Naomi was getting bigger, but that part of it was still hard for me. Rebecca and I never had our time. Naomi was always there, and she was right in the middle of her terrible twos, which could be difficult. When I tried to study, she always seemed to be crying, and she wouldn't stop. Honestly, it was really frustrating for me. I was twenty years old, and suddenly a stepfather, and I didn't have the slightest clue about babies, or about patience. So I sometimes went and stayed with Darwin at his new apartment.

I was so close to finishing school and making good on my NFL dreams, and I didn't want anything to get in the way of that. Rebecca and I figured it would be best if I got back into the dorms, so I could do what it took to finish strong and take the next step, not just for myself, but also for our family. And then, that summer, we'd move in together, and get married, and we'd always be together after that.

Around that time, we also had some trouble with Naomi's father, and I finally had to set him straight and tell him if he didn't start respecting Rebecca, and me, we'd have real problems. It all started to feel like a lot, maybe too much. I found myself worrying I might not be ready, and I couldn't hide my fears from Rebecca.

"Babe, I don't know, am I ready?" I asked.

"Really?" Rebecca said.

I felt awful, and I didn't say anything that would make it worse.

"Don't even play with me like that," she said. "If you say you don't want to do it, then don't. You go your way, and I'll go mine. I've got too much at stake here."

Immediately, I knew she was right. This wasn't just about
Rebecca and me. This was about Naomi, too, and the family we
were all forming together.

"I'm sorry," I said.

We took the night to cool off, and the next day, I came right
back.

"I don't know what I was thinking," I said. "I'm in. I'm in.
I'm in."

All of the football players were given manual labor jobs. The
team had hooked up with a local business, and we were supposed to do some work on campus for them. So that summer my
job was to basically pound stop signs into the ground. I was
working as much as I could, now that I was about to be married
with a kid, trying to earn enough to get by. I was a senior, and
the seniors often had dibs on the better jobs, and I was finally
getting paid a nice amount of money.

For our next job, about seven of us—four black guys and
three white guys—did some demolition on a dormitory. After
two weeks, our boss let the four black guys go, and the three
white guys stayed on all summer. It was obvious that racial discrimination was at play, and so I went to the coaches and com-
plained.

"They can choose whoever they want," the coaches said.

Again, I was so disappointed in the fact that the school didn't
take care of me that I whined about it for the rest of the summer. I was comparing my circumstances to rumors I'd heard
about star players getting preferential treatment at other, bigger
schools. The problem with my complaining was that I confused
it with action. I should have hunted far and wide for another
job, but instead, I just made excuses. I didn't work again for the
rest of the summer. And we were broke. I mean broke.

We couldn't afford a big party, but I wanted to get married

before football camp started up again, so Rebecca and I set our date for July 29, 1989, the day before my twenty-first birthday. We didn't have anything, so everybody we knew chipped in as much as they could, and our wedding was basically a big pot-luck dinner. It felt so cool to have everyone give back to us. Because I'd started to make a name for myself on the football team, we knew a lot of people on campus and in the community, and it was really special to be supported by them like that.

Rebecca was very active in our church and played music at services, but I'd kept some distance from organized religion after coming out of Maranatha. Still, it meant a great deal to us to be married by our pastor, since we'd first met at his church. Rebecca planned everything. I basically just rented a crisp white tux and showed up. I wore my practice shorts underneath my suit, and the words "Western Michigan #94" were visible through my white pants to anyone who looked long enough. I'd also experimented with my high-top fade and had a barber cut a part on a diagonal all the way through, from the front to the back. Everything left of the part was short, and everything to the right was long. It was a geometric wonder.

The ceremony was as good as I could have expected. As we exchanged our vows, two-year-old Naomi jumped up and grabbed onto my leg in the middle of everything. I held her for as long as I could to keep her calm, but when I had to put her down after we lit our unity candle, it was pure bedlam. She screamed as loud as she could for what seemed like an eternity. My brother, Marcelle, was my best man, and I had Darwin, JoNathan, Michael Lewis, and my childhood buddy Robert Blond as groomsmen. It was a full-on family affair. But when the ceremony was over, all I could think about was the bed-and-breakfast we had on reserve for the night in lieu of a real honeymoon. It was not easy getting Rebecca into my Chevy Nova because she was having such a wonderful time socializing with everyone. But she looked absolutely gorgeous, and I wanted to socialize with only her. Finally, I actually picked her up and put her in the car. All in all, it was a beautiful day.

I couldn't have been happier with Rebecca, and I loved Naomi and our little family, but as my senior year got under way, it was a very stressful time. I was so busy with the team that Rebecca and I would sometimes look at each other and wonder how we were going to do this, and if I could really graduate. Was it even possible? I started to see why athletes paid other people to do their papers for them. I never did, so I just submitted whatever I could, and then, whatever my grade was, that's what it was. I also had a bit of a hustle worked out. If I got a D in one class, I knew the A from my independent study in painting would keep my grade point average up enough to let me playing football. So I painted two or three really great paintings, and I held on to them. Then I purposefully made the rest of my paintings subpar. Because art is so subjective, my professors never actually told me they were bad. They just encouraged me to keep trying. I brought in one of my really terrible paintings and asked my professor how I could improve it, knowing all the while how and why it sucked. Then I made sure everything I showed them became progressively better. Toward the end of the semester, I handed in the three beautiful paintings and complimented the professor on how much his advice had helped me and made me a better artist. Totally flattered, and impressed with my improved artwork, my professors gave me an A both semesters.

As busy as I was, I certainly wasn't working. We had so little money that even though Rebecca and I lived together off campus, I didn't eat at home because I was scared to eat up all of

Rebecca and Naomi's food. I often snuck back into my old dormitory to eat, sometimes twice a day. This really nice older white guy headed up the kitchen, and he knew how much I was struggling.

"Terry, come on in," he said, smiling. "I know you want to eat."

"Thanks, man," I said, clapping his palm in a hearty handshake.

I was so appreciative whenever he waved me through. But it didn't always happen that way. One day, I was starving and late for practice when he stopped me.

"I can't do it today," he said. "I'm sorry."

He had snuck me in so many times that he was on the verge of getting in trouble. But even if he had to pull back on his kindness sometimes, he always found a way to let me back in again, and at the time, I was incredibly grateful. I knew I was breaking the rules, but at the same time, my sense of entitlement had turned me into a bit of a hustler, and the sad part is, I felt justified in getting over on others.

I was young and extremely immature. I'd had this vision that when I got married, things would just take care of themselves, but it wasn't happening. I had this great idea that I was going to make T-shirts and sell them. So I used the little bit of money I had to buy an airbrush.

"Why are you buying this thing?" Rebecca said. "You know, you'd better use it. Are you using it? Are you doing it?"

Of course I didn't follow through. I was always starting things like that, saying I was going to do them to get some money, and then I never did anything with them. I put Rebecca through a lot of stress.

At the time, credit card companies were handing out accounts like candy, and my whole mentality of entitlement meant that I'd charged up all of my cards. I had them all: American Express, Visa, MasterCard, Discover, and even a Sears card. They'd all since been halted, and I had no way to make even the minimum payments on them, so we had creditors calling the house constantly. On several occasions, there was a knock on the door of our apartment. When I answered, our upstairs neighbor was standing there looking sheepish.

"Hey, uh, Visa is on the line at my house, asking to talk to you," he said.

"Whoa, I'm sorry, man," I said. "We'll handle it."

But the real truth was, I didn't have any money coming in, and I wouldn't until I went pro. Looking back, I can see I was really very ignorant about the ways of the world, but at the time, I was young, and I was bound for glory, and I thought I knew everything. I think my attitude had a lot to do with growing up in a city like Flint, where everyone worked for General Motors, and the mentality was that GM was going to take care of us. GM was like our dad. We worked for the shop, and in return, they gave us a house, a car, whatever we needed. I had rejected that lifestyle because I didn't want to work for the shop, but I still had the mentality that someone owed me. That was part of how I'd grown up feeling so entitled, expecting my parents to give things to us, without ever really taking responsibility for them.

Usually, I dodged the calls, but one day I was around the house trying to study. I ended up on the phone with collections, and finally, I snapped.

"You don't pay your bills," he said.

"You know what, man," I said. "In a minute I'm going to be in the NFL, and you are still going to be calling people, begging for your little money. You probably don't make, what, eight dollars an hour, maybe, if that?"

Not that I was even making eight dollars an hour at the time, but you know.

"I'm going to be rich," I said. "And you're still going to be working there, and you're still going to be bothering people for their money."

Finally, Rebecca grabbed the phone out of my hand and hung it up.

A minute later, the phone rang again. Instead of being nervous about what this guy might say or do, I was so mad that I was ready to get back into it.

"Sir, you know what, I apologize," he said.

Well, now, this was the first time I'd ever had a bill collector call me back to say he was sorry, so maybe my rant had worked.

"Pay us when you can," he added before hanging up.

Even I was surprised to receive such kindness, but the stress I was under at the time was incredible, and I guess he could tell I was not in good shape.

Some days the phone rang and rang, and Naomi cried, and Rebecca looked at me like she was wondering what she had gotten herself into this time.

"We're gonna go pro, baby," I said. "And as soon as I go pro, all of these bills are going to be paid. So don't even worry."

"Okay, okay," she said, but she didn't sound convinced.

I was good at saying the right thing to keep Rebecca's anxiety at bay, but I wasn't always so good at convincing myself. After we'd been married for a few months, Rebecca got pregnant. I was excited to have a baby, but the thought of the cost and responsibility terrified me. There were times when Rebecca went off to work, and I watched Naomi, and I just sat there in a fog. On other days, when Naomi was with her babysitter, I started acting out in secret with pornography again. Every time, I felt guilty afterward, and I swore I'd never do it again, but somehow, I always did. I grew depressed, which made me even less able to get on top of our money problems and made things seem that much more overwhelming.

It didn't help that tensions were worse than ever between my football coaches and me, and I knew if I didn't hang on and make it through college, I'd jeopardize everything I'd worked so hard for since the seventh grade. It was a difficult season. And then, during a game, I got called to the sideline by one of my coaches. "Your wife's in the hospital," he said.

She'd had a miscarriage. I walked off the field and arrived at the hospital, sweaty and crying. "I'm sorry," I said. "I'm sorry. I'm sorry."

"What are you sorry about?" she said. "It's okay. You didn't have anything to do with it."

But in my heart, I knew I was being punished for my dark secret. Rebecca soon became pregnant again, and I was filled with fear. I tried my best to be good.

CHAPTER 8

DON'T YOU GIVE UP

THE PREVIOUS YEAR, EVEN WHEN I'D SOMETIMES felt discouraged by my football experience, we were playing so well that I got swept up in the excitement of winning. But this year, we had a terrible season, largely because we had a brilliant backup quarterback, who happened to be black. This was in the days when there hadn't been many black quarterbacks yet, so they benched him and played this little white freshman from Canada instead. It was not good. Our quarterback went in, led the nation in interceptions, and had a horrible time, but they stuck with him.

I'd always suspected there was racism at play on our team. From the beginning, my linebacker coach had told me that I wasn't smart enough to play linebacker (even though the NFL eventually thought I was intelligent enough to keep me there for six seasons). I noticed that he played all of the white guys in what they called the thinking man's spots, whereas I was forced to play a position that was about being a physical body. I knew I should have had a different position, because of my athleticism, but I also knew my ability to take a tremendous amount of physical pain was my ticket out, so I went with what I'd been given.

Most of the black players on the team were angry, but we didn't feel there was anything we could do. I later found out that the racial tension finally boiled over a few years after I left, and the black players actually had a sit-down strike, where they refused to even go out on the field because of the discrimination they felt.

What was happening on the football field at school primed me for a 1989 movie that shook me to the core: Spike Lee's *Do the Right Thing*. I probably saw that movie twenty times in the theater. I couldn't get enough. When *School Daze* had been released the year before, we'd had a midnight screening at school, and it was an event for all of the black students. This was even better. I'd never seen images so raw, so compelling, or so truthful. As *Star Wars* had done years earlier, it cemented my conviction that I was meant to be in film someday.

I wanted to write and direct my own movies, and Spike Lee was my hero. I found out that his aunt, Gloria Lee, worked at our college, and I tracked her down.

"Can I just paint a picture of Spike, and see if you like it, and if you do, maybe you could send it to him?" I asked.

"I've seen your work," she said. "If you make it, I will be sure he gets it."

I painted Spike's portrait, with all these headlines around him in the background. I used it as the final project for my independent study in painting, and then I had it framed. Gloria sent it off, and I was in suspense while I waited to see if he liked it. Well, a few weeks later, he sent back a book about the making of his new movie, *Mo' Better Blues,* with a personal note to Gloria from Spike: "Tell your student, Terry, thank you for the beautiful painting, and that I wish him luck."

That was like a lifeline for me. We were living in this basement apartment, really struggling, and yet I felt like I had touched Hollywood in some small way, and my life was never the same again. After that, I always knew I belonged in Hollywood, and I wouldn't be happy until I made it out there someday.

I certainly didn't want to be in Kalamazoo anymore. That was the beginning of a militant period for me, where I saw everything in racial terms, even though my wife was half white. I was big, I was black, and I was very aware of being treated like a threat. I felt like I could never get ahead as long as my coaches and bosses were discriminating against me. Of course, when I went back to Flint, and I saw the gangs and drugs and guys with six different kids by six different women, I was like, I can't end up over here with my own people when they're living like this, either.

I was young, and I was angry. Now I can see that my anger hurt me more than anyone else. There were times when it became a form of self-sabotage, because when I was mad, I was often blinded to the possibilities of my life. When I eventually realized this, I understood that I had to see what was actually open to me and do my best to achieve it. But at that time, I was experiencing my first political awakening, crude as it was. And I'm glad I went through that phase, because I think every young man needs to rebel to find his way—every young woman does, too—and this means cutting Mom's apron strings, and questioning Dad's lessons, questioning everything.

Rebecca was older than me, and way more mature, but she was always patient with me, and my growing pains, even when she became pregnant again not long after her first miscarriage, and she really needed me to grow up. She had graduated beauty school with all of the awards, and she'd gotten a job at Regis, a hair place at the mall. It was a great job, and they were paying her well. Finally, it seemed like an end to our worries might be in sight. And then, just as she'd started to attract a lot of clients, and she was about to get a raise, one of her friends opened a shop and asked Rebecca to go work for her. I was already feeling guilty enough about the fact that I was playing football, which meant I couldn't make any money. And then she jumped ship from this really great job to her friend's salon and ended up making very little. "Becky, uh, you do know we have nothing, right?" I said.

"I've got to help my friend," she said. "I've got to do this."

So then we were even broker than we had been, which I hadn't even thought was possible. With another baby on the way, I had to make it to the pros.

I couldn't wait for my football dream to come true and take me all the way to the NFL. But as hard as I'd worked, and as ready as I felt, it wasn't going to be easy. Our daughter Azriel was born on November 13, 1990, in Kalamazoo, Michigan. And so now we were down in our basement apartment with Naomi climbing all over, and with little bitty Azi sitting in her chair, and Rebecca and I just trying to make it.

I threw everything I had into my final season of college football. The school held what were called pro days, when NFL scouts came and talked to the most celebrated players. A few scouts had sat me down for meetings that fall, but no one ever called me back to follow up. I was sure I was going to fight my way into the NFL, but this lack of serious attention was making me nervous, especially because I'd gotten some light from the pros after our championship, and now it felt like the momentum had slowed, just when I needed it to pick up. My big thing was that I had to make it to the NFL Combine in February. During two and a half days in Indianapolis, representatives from all of the NFL teams would get a look at the best up-and-coming college players. And it was unclear if I was going to be there or not.

My deteriorating relationship with my coaches wasn't helping. We were doing a drill on the field during practice when another player began doing some dirty stuff, and I fought back. The coach jumped up on me and started screaming.

"Terry, what are you doing?"

"I was protecting myself," I said.

"Get off the field. Go in the locker room. Take a shower. You're done."

Like I said, I'd believed there was a difference between the way the coaches treated the white players and the way they treated the black players, and in my mind, this was just one more example. Once you see your world in those terms, everything in your line of vision becomes a discriminatory situation. At the time, I saw them as being out to get me. Now, I believe my bad attitude had poisoned our relationship. I was ready to storm off the field, but then it hit me: *I may lose my scholarship if I leave this practice.*

"No, if I leave this field, you're going to try to take my scholarship," I said. "I'm going to stay right here. You're going to coach, and I'm going to play, and that's the way it's going to be."

With my mind-set the way it was then, I felt like I'd had no choice but to react the way I did. Of course, as I would discover years later, we always have a choice. But, at the time, it was too late. They were done with me, and I was done with them. They played me because I was still one of the best guys on the field, but I treated every word they said to me with disdain.

"You'd better be appreciative," my coach said.

"Wait a minute," I said. "Why aren't *you* appreciative? *You* should be thanking *me*."

He was so mad he looked ready to have a heart attack. But I didn't care how much they hated me. My anger had taken over.

Finally, I got a call from Ronny Jones, the linebacker coach for the Los Angeles Rams. He came to town and took me out to dinner.

"Terry, what is the deal with your coaches on your team?" he said.

"What do you mean?"

"I called everybody, and they said they didn't know where you were," he said. "They said they have no contact with you."

I froze right there, seated across from him at the table.

"They know exactly where I am," I said. "I live off campus, but they have my address right there in their files."

"They tried to say they had no idea where you were," he said. "They were literally saying, 'We don't know, and we don't care.' It took me forever to find you."

It turned out I'd had several scouts from NFL teams try to come see me in the previous weeks, but the coach's office hadn't given them my address. I'd finished playing for the university at this point, but I still had to get through about four months of school, and my relationship with the coaches was at an all-time low.

After the season was over, we had this big banquet where they honored the players of the year. I knew I'd had a good year. The pro scouts I'd met with had all been talking about what was going to happen, how good I was going to be. And yet I was completely ignored at the banquet. Even though I'd had so much tension with my coaches, I'd played my heart out for my chance to play in the League. I wanted them to recognize my

ability, but I'm sure they saw things I couldn't see in myself at
the time. I had become a brat.

When they ignored me at that banquet, very few moments
in my life have ever been as painful. The room was decorated
with photographs of all the graduating seniors, and as I stalked
out at the end of the evening, I grabbed mine and took it with
me. A friend of mine gave me a ride home, and as I sat in his car
with this big cardboard photo on my lap, my anger raged inside
of me until I couldn't stand it anymore. I opened his car window
and threw my picture out into the night. I'd lost respect for my
coaches and the way the college football franchise was run long
ago, but I'd had to play nice as long as my livelihood and my
future depended on my place on the team. Now that school was
over, I was done.

Looking back at that time in my life, now that everything
isn't so emotionally charged, and I have the advantage of distance, I know that I should have had a better attitude, and if I'd
been able to be more positive, my coaches probably would have
treated me with more respect. When I was writing this book, I
first portrayed myself as a victim in my descriptions of my time
at school, without even realizing it. I glossed over my own faults
while putting all of the blame on my coaches. After my flawed
perspective was pointed out to me, I realized I was still angry.
What I've discovered as I've worked to finally grow up and become a better person, while making peace with my past, is that
anger can trick us. If we don't let our anger go naturally, it can
become an offense we hold on to that blinds us, clouding our
ability to see our own behavior clearly and causing us to become
helpless. It's like removing our hands from the wheel of our
own life, and letting whoever offended us drive, while we sit
meekly in the passenger seat, holding the offense in our lap. I'd

been able to see this in all of the other areas of my life, except for my time at Western Michigan, until only recently. Even now, as I'm wrapping up this book, I have to let go of whatever offends me and get control of the wheel—and, finally, drive my own life. But, at the time, I was just holding on as best as I could.

When I got home from the banquet at the end of my senior year, I climbed into bed with Rebecca. We had this old, used bed, and all of the springs had gone out of the middle, so it was sloped like a canoe. I fell into the middle of our sagging, lumpy mattress, and I looked around. The house was a mess. We were broke.

"I'm done," I said. "I'm done. I guess maybe I can go to art school."

"No, don't you give up," she said. "Don't give up on this football dream of yours. This was your dream."

"I know, but I can't take it anymore. All of this rejection. All of these guys. I can't take it. I don't want to do it anymore. I'm through."

"Honey, just give it a day," she said.

Literally the next day, I received my invitation to the Combine. When the papers came in the mail, I held them up triumphantly.

"Look at this, Becky," I said, reading the cover letter. "'You have been invited to the National Football League Combine in Indianapolis, Indiana.'"

I looked up at her. "I'm going to the Combine! I'm going! I'm going!"

She just stood there beaming at me. She'd known it was going to happen all along, and she hadn't let me give up, even when I was at my lowest.

I got on a plane for Indianapolis, and I was so excited. This was the event where all of the college players I'd heard about were brought together in preparation for the draft. On day one, it was all of the linebackers, and then, on the next day, it was the running backs, and so on.

As happy as I was to be there, the process was definitely uncomfortable. We were given a T-shirt with a number on it, and then we were paraded around in front of the scouts, like meat, so they could see our structure.

"Take your shirts off," a man shouted.

I did as I was told, feeling like I was at a slave auction, although it was the same treatment for all of us—white, black, and everyone in between.

"Turn to the front," he said. "Turn to the back."

They had a dentist examine our teeth. They gave us all of these tests, and they had us do drills and scrimmages against one another. The whole time, I was so nervous, and all I could think was: *I've got to do a good job. I've got to do a good job.*

I performed very, very well—so well that I was ranked according to my athletic ability as fifth in the nation for inside linebacker, which I'd never played before because it was one of the positions my college coach had felt was a smart man's spot, and so he'd had me play defensive end instead. Now the NFL coaches were saying this was the position I should be playing, and not only that, but I was ranked above all of these other players who'd held that position in college.

"You should have never been playing this position," the coaches said. "Why in the world did they have you down there?"

I knew I was doing well, and then, as I used to do, I got a little cocky. That's how I was back then: from one extreme to the other, from the depths of depression to being so giddy with delight it was unrealistic. Well, it was only February, and I had to wait until the draft in April to see if my confidence was justified or not.

———

FINALLY, THE NFL DRAFT WAS COMING UP ON APRIL 22, 1991. This was a week before my senior year ended, but I loaded up a truck without finishing school or earning a degree, and we moved. Rebecca and I had a nice little apartment set up, and it would have made more sense to stay there until I went pro and found out where my new team was located.

"Why are we leaving now?" Rebecca said. "Why don't we see where you go?"

"I can't," I said. "We've just got to get out of here."

It wasn't a logical assessment of the situation, but I was so angry I couldn't stand to be around that school anymore. I couldn't stand to be in Kalamazoo, either. This will tell you just how much I wanted to go: In order to get out of Kalamazoo as soon as possible, and given the fact that we had no money and a mountain of debt, Rebecca and I actually returned to Flint and moved in with my mother and father. Not my ideal living situation, or theirs. And, on top of that, I had twelve credits left in order to complete my college education, and I never finished.

With no college degree, no job prospects, no place to live, and no money, my entire future was once again riding on what I'd been able to accomplish on the football field. And now my prospects also included that of my family: Rebecca, Naomi, and our new baby, Azriel. This was a lot of pressure, but I was more confident than I'd ever been before, coming off of my scholarship experience, and the conversations I'd had with pro scouts, and my trip to the Combine.

I was so sure there was a place in the NFL for me that I had a big barbecue on Draft Day and invited all of my family and old friends from Flint to come over. On Sunday morning, people started arriving, and I started barbecuing. We spent the early part of the day eating and hanging around, anticipating the good news. The draft started at noon. I didn't necessarily expect to get picked in the first round, but I figured my new team would call me early in the draft to give me the good news. Everyone would be there, and it would be this great, big celebration.

"You know, I might get drafted in the second round," I said to whoever would listen. "Or maybe the fifth."

Or maybe not.

We waited all day. People came and went, and still there was no phone call. By mid-afternoon, I knew that the first six or seven rounds were over, and clearly I had not been drafted yet. But that was okay. There were twelve rounds in total over two days, which left plenty of opportunities for me.

Finally, the phone rang. Everyone made room for me, and I answered.

"This is the Dallas Cowboys," a man's voice said.

"Yeah!" I said. I was literally cheering, I was so happy. The Dallas Cowboys was my favorite team growing up. It was a dream come true to play for them.

"Hey, man, I'm just kidding," the man said.

What?! It took me a minute to process what was happening, and then I realized that I recognized the voice on the other end of the line: Marcelle.

"I could kill you right now," I said.

Without another word, I hung up on him. I couldn't believe he'd done that to me. It was the meanest trick anyone had ever played on me, and it was literally several weeks before I was able to talk to him again.

By this point, it was late in the afternoon, and the day had definitely lost its luster. Everyone went home, and the party was finished. The first day of the draft passed without a call. I woke up early the next day and continued to wait by the phone. Hours passed. At this point, it was three or four in the afternoon, and it appeared my greatest fear had come true. The NFL didn't want me. It was over.

"I didn't get drafted," I said, collapsing in a heap on the stairs. I turned around and put my face down, and I just cried, I mean real tears and sobs.

"I didn't do it," I said. "I didn't do it. I failed."

"Terry," Rebecca said. "What are you doing? Listen, if you were supposed to do this, you are going to do it. You did the whole walk-on thing in college, and you can do it again. I don't care if you have to try out. Or if you have to go free agent, that's what you're going to do. If this is your dream, it's yours. God did not take you this far to leave you here, so you get yourself together, and understand that this is not the end, ever."

I looked at her. She had shaken me up, but in a good way. She was right.

"I know," I said, wiping away my tears.

"Now stop it, and understand there is something bigger for you. Get yourself together right now, and we're gonna believe the best is yet to come, okay?"

"I know," I said, through the last of my tears. "I know."

I felt like I was done, but I knew she was right. And if she still believed in me, then I had to find a way to believe in myself.

Rebecca and my mother left for the grocery store. The phone rang. I didn't even notice. At this point, I was past caring. So my sister picked up the phone.

"Terry," Micki said.

I looked up, but I was beyond even daring to hope.

"I think it's the LA Rams," she said.

Oh, no, you are not going to play me a second time, Marcelle, not today.

"Is this something Marcelle planted?" I said.

She shook her head. As I walked toward her, she held out the phone.

"If this is Marcelle again, I'm going to drive over there, and we're going to have to fight over this one."

Finally, I took the phone, too nervous to be excited.

"Hey, this is Ronny Jones from the Los Angeles Rams. I wanted to let you know that you were just selected in the eleventh round of the NFL draft by the LA Rams. I want to say congratulations, and we want you on a plane tomorrow."

IT WAS SO GOOD. Just like with my football scholarship, I had thought it was over, but it was not over.

"Are you serious?" I said. "Really? Thank you, Mr. Jones."

Just as I hung up the phone, Rebecca came home.

"Hey, babe, I got drafted!"

She ran over and hugged me, and we started screaming. SCREAMING.

"Oh my God, I'm going to have a heart attack," Trish said.

We cheered, and celebrated, and cheered some more. IT WAS SO GOOD. I hadn't been drafted until almost the lowest round. There were only twelve rounds at the time, and they don't even have that many now. These days, they only go to eight. But I didn't care. All that mattered was it had happened.

Just like I'd gotten my scholarship, in the nick of time, I'd slid into the NFL right at the last moment. But in both cases, they'd let me in, and as far as I was concerned, that's all I needed. They had given me just enough recognition and encouragement, and I was going to hold on to it. This is where being extreme has actually always worked in my favor. The lows are low, yes, but all I need is the littlest yes, and I will take it all the way. That's how I've always been.

"Thank you," I said. "Thank you so much for shaking me out of that."

"Aw, I knew you could do it, Boo Boo," Rebecca said.

We hugged and hugged, while my mom and sister cheered. After everything we'd already been through in our short marriage, we were more than ready for a little good news and the hope of an even better tomorrow. After the devastation of the miscarriage, and the money problems, and the stress, to then experience the joy of having another baby and seeing my career take off like this made me feel like I had a chance after all.

The next day, I got on a plane for Orange County. I signed a contract with the Los Angeles Rams for $75,000, which seemed like big money. But what many people don't know is that NFL player contracts are game-to-game. There's no guaranteed salary. Once again, my money could be taken away from me at any time, if I got cut.

Because I'd been putting off paying our bills until I got signed, and I still couldn't handle my finances, we had all new money problems now. For starters, my paycheck wasn't as big as I'd thought it would be. And I still didn't spend the money we did have on paying the bills. I was all about looking good. I was all about feeling good. I was all about indulging. I was all about avoiding any type of pain. If I felt stressed or unhappy, my solution was to go buy something.

Rebecca was much smarter than I was about this stuff, but she tended to go along with me. I was the kind of type A force of nature that wouldn't take no for an answer. I had learned that I could get what I wanted if I kept pushing. And by this point, I could talk a really good game about how our life was going to be, and how we were going to be so much richer. In the meantime, we just barely kept ourselves afloat.

CHAPTER 9

NO WIVES ALLOWED

'D BEEN SHOCKED TO LEARN THAT RIGHT AFTER YOU'RE drafted you report to the team immediately, and now I was on a flight bound for John Wayne Airport in Orange County, after a connecting flight to Chicago. I could barely contain my excitement. *I made it. I am on an NFL football team.* The team's first-round draft pick, Todd Lyght, had been a cornerback at Notre Dame, but in a strange coincidence, he'd attended high school at Flint's Powers Catholic. I noticed him on my flight, but I was pretty sure he didn't have any idea who I was. I thought back to how I'd written all of those letters to different powerhouse football programs, and Notre Dame was definitely on the list. I looked at him as he sat in front of me, sizing him up after every air bump, wondering what exactly made him worth millions of dollars more than me. I scanned the back of his head for any sign of weakness, or any noticeable chink in his armor, so I could somehow increase my value in my own mind. It didn't matter that we didn't play the same position, that we both played defense, or that we were on the same team. To me, he was a threat. I knew I had to make an impact immediately if I was going to stay in the NFL. I wanted no one to impress the team more than I did. I'd finally gotten my foot in the door of my dream, and I was going to do whatever it took to remain there. He fell asleep, and so I finally looked away, realizing I'd have to wait to find out what he was made of. My nerves were on edge as I thought about every possible scenario before we'd even landed. *What if they don't like me? What if I'm not good enough? What will I do if this doesn't work out?*

A van with a driver picked me up at the airport, but Todd was whisked away by someone else. By mid-afternoon, I arrived at Ram Park in Anaheim. The three-hour time difference from Michigan to California was significant, because it seemed like almost no time had passed during my flight. The facility looked like an old, converted elementary school. Everything was immaculate and orderly. I met the team's equipment manager, Don Hewitt, who greeted me like an old friend. He knew how special the moment was for every new draftee who walked through the door.

I actually gasped when I walked into the locker room for the first time. The Rams' blue and gold team colors were everywhere: a Los Angeles Rams logo was emblazoned on the blue carpet, and the wide gold lockers doubled as seats when players turned to face the center of the room. A bag was waiting for me, containing my practice grays, shorts, and a gray shirt—"LA Rams" printed on the front of each—as well as my turf shoes. My locker had been marked with a piece of athletic tape, with "Crews" written on it in Magic Marker. As I surveyed the empty room, I saw the names of superstars written on the other lockers: #91 Kevin Greene, #83 Flipper Anderson, and #11 Jim Everett. Also a member of the team at that time was future wrestling superstar Bill Goldberg.

I went out for a look at the practice field: acres and acres of beautifully manicured grass, with white chalk lines signifying yard markers. As I passed outside to the field, I noticed players working out in the covered outdoor weight room. I tried my best not to stare as I sized up each and every one of them, quickly looking away when they caught my eye. It was so much to take in, and I was exhausted. When I was dropped off at my new home, an Oakwood temporary apartment near Buena Park, I collapsed with relief.

I was just in heaven. I'd made it to Orange County, and as far as I was concerned, that was Hollywood. While we were still in mini-camp, our team's superstar player, Todd Lyght, and his friend, Pat Terrell, decided to go up to LA for Queen Latifah's birthday party. I wanted to go so badly, and when they invited me to join them, that was it for me.

We got in the car, and we started driving, and driving, and driving. Now, I'd joined the LA Rams thinking there would be movies shooting right down the street, not realizing that we were actually based in Orange County. I was in shock when we drove for two hours before we finally rolled up to the Palladium in Hollywood.

Todd and Pat were dressed up, but I couldn't afford nice clothes, so I was wearing these denim overalls, which was the cool look back in the day. I still had my high-top fade, and I was feeling all right. Only there was a dress code, and the bodyguard wouldn't let me into the club. Todd was the first-round pick for the Rams that year, and everyone knew him, so he decided he was going to play on that.

"Please, man, just let my guy in," Todd said.

Meanwhile, I pulled out my NFL Players Association card, and held it up, as if that was going to do something for me. The bouncer actually laughed at me.

Okay, so that's not how it's done, I thought.

The bouncer finally let us in, no thanks to me, but I was floating. *This is LA,* I thought. *This is the real deal.* It was packed. And then I looked around, and it got even better: Queen Latifah, Kid 'n Play, Kadeem Hardison from *A Different World.*

We were able to go into the VIP section, and I saw none other than Prince sitting there with a bodyguard on either side of him. *I've got to meet Prince. I've just got to meet him. I don't know when I'll get another chance, and there's no way I'm going to be in LA and not make it happen.* I approached his table, and his bodyguards stood up and gave me a warning look. I was big, but they were bigger than me.

"Hey, guys, how you doing?" I said. "Terry Crews, LA Rams."

They looked at me like: *Who is this joker?* I mean, it was just terrible.

"Excuse me, excuse me, Prince, how you doing?" I said, sticking my hand out. "I'm Terry Crews with the Los Angeles Rams."

"Hey, nice to meet you," he said, taking my hand. "Good to see you."

And then I didn't know what else to do. I just stood there and looked at him. "You're Prince," I said.

I mean, I was that idiot. I didn't know what else to say.

"Yes, yes, good to see you," he said.

"All right, see you later," I said.

I flashed two thumbs up to the bodyguards and then turned and walked away. At first I felt like I'd messed it up, but then I was like: *I met Prince.* And then I met Wesley Snipes, who was just coming off *New Jack City.*

"Man, you are awesome," I said, shaking his hand.

Yes, I was that guy, telling everyone how great they were. I'm sure they all looked at me like: *Yeah, who is this guy? What planet is he from?* But nothing could bring me down. *This is Hollywood. This is so cool. It's the best thing ever.*

I was on a high the whole drive back to Orange County. The people I'd listened to back in Flint, and the stars I'd seen when I went to the movies in college, they were real. I'd met them. It was so surreal.

Back in my apartment, I lay in bed and picked up the phone.

"Becky, I'm in LA," I said. "We are doing it. We are doing it."

"Okay, that's cool, honey," she said. "That's cool."

It was cool. I couldn't sleep. I was too excited.

By the time camp finally rolled around, I was ready to hit something and somebody. We checked into the University of California, Irvine. I was placed in a dormitory with three other roommates and one mission: Don't get cut. I was given a play-book the size of the phonebook. It was so full of jargon and obscure terminology, it might as well have been written in Spanish.

My first few days in camp, I knew I had to get noticed, and fast, or else I would fade into the sea of overripe Rams jerseys just waiting to be plucked and thrown out. My strategy was to fight. I perceived any slight—mistaken or intentional—as war. A small shove after the whistle, a running back who got up after a tackle with a kick, even any little bit of trash talk, was a reason to start something. Not that I was actually angry, but I proved I was a pretty capable actor back then, what with the way I hammed it up in my altercations.

I was soon known as a scrapper. Head Coach John Robinson yelled at me to cut it out every time I started swinging on my teammates, but when he walked away, I caught the faintest smirk on his face. He liked it, and he liked me. That's all I needed to know. Things were off to a good start, and it was a huge relief.

The reality of life on the team still took some getting used to, though. One of the strangest sights I can remember ever seeing happened during our lunch between practices on one of our two-a-days, when we had practice twice in one day. The police showed up in the cafeteria with one of the biggest men I'd ever seen, handcuffed and looking sullen. The officers brought him over to the food line, uncuffed him, and let him go. I asked someone what all this was about, and he told me the guy was accused of sexually assaulting a woman who'd been babysitting his kids. I had no idea whether this was true or not, but having seen those cuffs come off, I decided my little fight strategy was not going to involve this guy.

One of my roommates was cut, but I made it through camp. I received encouraging words from some of the executives and coaches, and I felt like I was going to make it. I moved back into Oakwood and waited the week for the season to start, keeping Rebecca up on what was happening by phone. Amazingly, my habit of acting out with pornography disappeared during this time because I didn't want any guilt to get in the way of me making the team. I even got to have my college number—#94— and I felt things were on track. I was going to make it.

Then the coach wanted to see me. This was never good.

He called me into his office and told me they were going to cut me. I couldn't believe it. This had to be a joke. I had been the victim of tons of hazing during the camp—singing in the cafeteria, being taped to a goalpost, and having food smeared in my high-top fade—and the veterans on the team had even snuck into my dorm room and sprayed a fire extinguisher all over my clothes and me in the middle of the night. Surely I couldn't have gone this far just to be sent home.

The reality was, yes, he had to cut me. But. He was bringing me back as part of the practice squad. I breathed a sigh of relief. It was much less money, but I wasn't going home. I was still a member of the team. The coach even took the unprecedented step of letting me travel with the squad as a practice squad player. I was honored, and happy, and I quickly relieved Rebecca with the (mostly) good news. Two weeks into my stint on the practice squad, a player was hurt, and I was activated to the active roster. Rebecca and the kids immediately came out to Anaheim to be with me. My dream had come true.

At first, every moment in the NFL was magic: *I can't believe I'm in camp! I can't believe I'm in the Rams locker room! I can't believe I'm in a football stadium!* If I'd spent my youth wondering what a man was, and when I would be one, there was no doubt I was among men now. These were the men, of the men, of the men.

That didn't last, though. There were drugs in the locker room. And I was thinking, *No, that's not good. That's not what I want to see.* And then I got invited to a night out with some of my teammates, and one of them pulled me aside. "Man, you know, it's men only, no wives," he said. "No wives allowed. It's a guy thing."

Without even thinking about it, I went home and told Rebecca that I was going out with just the guys. She knew she could trust me, and that I wanted to become friends with my new teammates, so she didn't make a fuss about it. I showed up to meet the guys, and it was a big free-for-all with these other girls. *They said no wives,* I thought. *But I guess they didn't mean no girls.* And, again, I thought: *Nah, nah, that's not what I want to see. That's not what I'm talking about.*

I was scared to say anything to the guys about what they were doing because, you know, I'm human, and I wanted them to like me. I was scared to tell my wife what they were up to when they weren't around their wives, and for a long time I didn't, because I knew she'd never let me out again.

It was always something. One night, we were in Atlanta, and I didn't want to sit alone in my hotel room, so I went out with a bunch of the other players before a game. I got into the back of someone's car, and I couldn't believe what I saw.

"What is this, man?" I said. "There's a gun in here."

They acted like it was nothing. So, again, I didn't say anything. Of course, we got pulled over. One of the guys in the front seat reached back and handed me the gun.

"Here, put this in the back!" he said. "Put this in the back!"

I wasn't into this at all. This was the kind of craziness that had made me fight so hard to get out of Flint. But I didn't exactly have a choice at that point, so I took the gun, and I put it under the seat. *I'm going to jail,* I thought. *I'm going to jail. Just because I wanted to not sit in my hotel room.*

It got worse. As the cop approached the open window, I couldn't believe what came out of the driver's mouth.

"Man, why are you pulling me over?" he said.

"Would you shut your mouth?" I whispered from the back-seat.

When the cop went to write us a ticket, I let the driver have it.

"If you give him one more word, I'm gonna hit you in the back of the head," I said. "Brother, you are not taking me to jail with your attitude. I'm not doing it."

And that was one of the tame stories. It got to where I

dreaded having one of the other guys say, "Come hang out with me, man."

The first time we traveled to New York City, I couldn't believe I'd made it to the big city, the center of so much art and culture I'd always admired. The coaches told another player and me that we weren't playing the next day, so we were free to relax. I was disappointed not to play, but I was excited to see New York City.

"Come hang out with me, man," the other guy said.

I should have known better, but the NFL world was still so new and exhilarating for me. *Wow, I get to hang out with a football player in New York,* I thought. *This is going to be amazing.* Actually, it was awful. This guy grabbed a bunch of drugs and a couple of hookers, hailed a cab, and had the driver take him around in circles while he was doing his business. My job was to make sure he made it back to our hotel. Meanwhile, I stood on the corner, miserable. *Dude, I just want to go home,* I thought. But I didn't know where we were, or how to get back to our hotel.

Plus, I knew if I left him on his own, I would never hear the end of it from the other guys on our team. It's a shame dynamic with guys. That's why I've always said, if there's a pack of four guys, even four really good guys, something stupid is about to happen. Because no one wants to seem weak in front of the other guys, and so they will do anything, anything, just to prove they'll do it. That's why we need that female energy around to get us to stop and think about what we're doing. Otherwise, we will go right off the ledge, and everybody's too scared to stop it.

Whenever we arrived in a new city for a game, the first stop was always a strip club. Even though I had my pornography issue, I couldn't handle seeing women in that way live. Even back then, I understood that the dynamic of pornography was to get men to see women as objects, which distanced me from the women enough to allow me to deny their humanity, and somehow made it manageable for me, even though I knew it wasn't good. If we were together in the same room, I saw them as people, and I couldn't enjoy it. When I walked into a strip club, I knew I was seeing somebody's sister, somebody's mother, somebody's daughter. After our first strip club outing, I realized: *Man, I can't do this. This is not me. I don't want to do this.* And so I sat outside many a strip club while my teammates were inside. It was hard because I didn't want to be there, but just like in college, I didn't want to be alone, either. I needed community, and I wanted to be with my crew. I could see how a person's core values would get chipped away under such circumstances, and I tried to hold on to mine.

My disillusionment with my teammates was one thing. I liked them as people. I just didn't want to behave that way myself. The reality check I received from the NFL was another thing, and just like with college football, I was soon disappointed. I saw so much dirty stuff. My friend Anthony's coaches told him they really wanted him to play in the next day's game. He resisted because his knee was bothering him, but they persisted, saying he was the future of the franchise. Well, they didn't play him once, not until the last two minutes, when they put him in for one play. When they cut him from the team the next day, he protested because he was hurt. They told him they had footage of him playing the day before, so he couldn't be injured. They took his money and sent him away. It was the most brutal thing imaginable.

Not to mention another fact I soon realized: The individual teams didn't really matter because all of the money went to the league anyhow. Let's just say that my whole opinion of everything changed very quickly.

But there I was, among the most elite athletes in the world, and, of course, I wanted to do everything I could to prove I belonged. And I wanted to take my career in the NFL as far as I possibly could. I certainly wasn't going back to Flint. This was just the beginning for me. And, besides, I had to keep playing because our money problems were only getting worse. I didn't end up playing in a game until my second year on the Rams, which meant we had to live on $75,000 for that whole time. That would have been totally fine, except for all of the debt I'd accumulated, and the fact that I insisted on living like I was earning a lot more than I was. On top of that, we had a dismal year, ending up with a 3-win, 13-loss record. Not good, to say the least.

My second year on the team, John Robinson and the coaching staff who'd drafted me were fired. Suddenly, I had to prove myself to our new coach, Chuck Knox, and his team of assistants. I was low on the totem pole to begin with, and the new coaches came in planning to make a ton of changes, which did not bode well for me. And then I came head-to-head with one of the coaches. He berated me. He dogged me out. He belittled me in every way imaginable. One time, he got a colonoscopy, and he privately showed me the pictures.

"Look at that, you ever see a pucker like that?" he said.

"Why are you showing me that?" I said, trying to look away.

He kept trying to get my attention. "Hey, Tyrone," he said. "Hey."

"No, my name is Terry."

"I like Tyrone. I'm going to call you Tyrone."

I was seething, but I let it go. *He's not going to break me,* I thought. I wondered if maybe it was like that movie *An Officer and a Gentleman,* where they tried to break Richard Gere's character until he found the magic way to get out from under them.

Only I couldn't see an end in sight, and nothing I did helped, not even when I played hard and made things happen on the field.

One day we were in practice, looking over footage from the last game, and he zipped right through the film of me. That time, the other players noticed.

"Hey, hey, hey, Terry just got an interception," said Kevin Greene, the star linebacker at the time.

"Ah, it doesn't matter," the coach said. "He's not going to be here."

I couldn't hide how mad I was. "What is that?" I said.

"You know what?" the coach said to me. "You sucker, you're going to end up with an apple and a bus ticket. That's it. You can't play. The only reason you're here is because somebody up there likes you. But I don't care about you."

He made me feel so small, but I was such a pleaser that I wanted him to like me, even though anyone could have told me there was nothing I could do to make things right with him. I took his abuse because I was so scared of losing my place on the team. And then he cut me at the end of the season anyhow. At first, I actually thought that maybe this was just another one of his tricks. But it wasn't.

It started to eat at me that I'd never stood up for myself and told him that the way he was talking to me was unacceptable. He had gotten inside my head in the worst possible way and made me feel so low. Now I didn't have a place on the team, and I didn't even have my self-respect. Honestly, that was the closest I've ever come to killing someone. I plotted the whole thing out, fantasizing about how I would wait for him to come outside after practice. Obviously, I never would have taken it that far, but it got so dark for a time that I felt like I could have done it.

CHAPTER 10

IT'S NOT OVER

Y AGENT WAS UPBEAT, SAYING HE WAS GOING to try to get me on another team. There was nothing to do but wait. We'd spent the little bit of money I'd been given, so we were broke, and I kept thinking about all of the things I should have done differently, but it was too late for any of that now. We sat in our tiny apartment, and every little thing set me off. I yelled at Rebecca. I yelled at the kids. I said things to Rebecca she didn't deserve. I definitely was not nice.

I felt such immense pain and pressure pushing down on me, and I wanted to give up. I wanted everyone to leave me alone. Not that it helped when people did leave us alone. I might not have wanted to run wild through the streets with my teammates, but I'd loved that feeling of being a part of a team, and I still wanted to hang out with the other players. Well, when we were cut, we called people who had been our friends the week before, and they didn't call us back. I got it. We weren't on the team anymore, and they were, and they felt uncomfortable. But it was rough. We still went to the same restaurants and grocery stores, and our kids still went to the same schools, but we were out, and they were in, simple as that.

Finally, we returned to Flint and moved back in with my parents. The dynamic was problematic from the start. My sister, Micki, was in high school now, and she was always telling me how things should be. We got into a lot of fights. "You know, I'm a grown man with a family," I said, not getting that the funny thing is, grown men with families shouldn't move back in with their mothers, except under the most dire circumstances. Here I was, acting like the whole world was my hotel.

Trish came in and inevitably took sides.

"Well, your sister's right," Trish said.

I was angry all of the time and scared about what might come next.

Hard to believe I could be dumber than I already was, but things got worse. Right before the Rams cut me, they gave me a $40,000 signing bonus to come back to the team for a second season, and I went and bought a Nissan Pathfinder, which was the hottest car back then. Never mind that we didn't have a place to live, and we were staying with my parents, so long as I had a nice car. Rebecca had been very supportive, but she couldn't keep quiet this time.

"Couldn't we use that money to buy a small house, and maybe live there, and we'll just keep the car that we have?" she said. "Or shouldn't we get an apartment?"

"Oh, no, no, I can't do that," I said.

I cringe thinking about it now. I was literally outside of my parents' house, washing my new car, while my wife and two kids were inside. But at the time, I just wanted what I wanted, and I didn't think about how it was for anyone else.

Now that I'd been cut, all I had was that car. And the car payments.

Oh, snap, how are we going to do this? I thought.

Finally, in 1993, the Green Bay Packers signed me. I went up there to join the team. But this wasn't quite the solution I'd hoped it would be. The season started up, and I didn't play. This meant I wasn't getting paid. They gave me $200 a week to work out, and that was it. I had spent all of the money I had on the car, and clothes, and going out to eat, so I had no money, and the bills were piling up, and the credit cards were not getting paid, and creditors were once again calling all of the time. I couldn't afford to make payments on the Pathfinder anymore, and soon there were repo men looking for me to take the car back. At least we were lucky enough that my parents let Rebecca and the kids stay on at their house in Flint.

I spent all of that off-season in a motel room in Green Bay. It was cold and gray. I was still seething about my old Rams coach. I was trying as hard as I could with the Packers, but making the team was a long shot. Nothing was working out the way I'd wanted it to, and my wife and kids were far away.

So, again, as happened during stressful times, I acted out. I rented a video machine and adult movies to play in the motel room. There were times I got magazines from the liquor store. When I went in, the clerk would ask what number I was, because the only black people in Green Bay at the time were on the football team. I did all of this without a car, walking to the video and liquor stores after I was done with workouts. Sometimes I'd work out in the morning, play dominoes with my teammates at our motel, then work out again in the afternoon, out of boredom, and then act out with pornography at night. In the strangest way, I felt like I deserved it. In particular, on Friday nights, after a long week of training and working out, the guys went out to bars and drank. Instead, I just found some porn and went back to my room. I treated it like my reward for a long week in Green Bay. This was the same pattern I'd had in college, and one I would have well into the years when I'd launched a successful entertainment career.

Partway into the season, a teacher invited some players to her classroom in Milwaukee to talk to the kids. Well, we pretended it was for the kids, but we really just wanted out of our motel. We went and, compared to Green Bay, Milwaukee felt like New York City. Before the other players and I left, the teacher pulled me aside.

"Anytime you want to come see the city, you know, whatever," she said.

And then she sent me a picture of her, with myself and another player from the team. Rebecca was visiting, and she saw the picture.

"I don't like her," she said. "Something's up with her."

"There's nothing wrong with her," I said.

"I don't like her."

"I don't know," I said. "I don't know."

Yeah, wife always knows, that's the deal.

Green Bay in the early spring is *not* a tourist destination. I was going stir-crazy. So I went to Milwaukee to see the teacher. She showed me around, and then she set up this whole picnic.

Uh.

I felt nervous, but I didn't want to be back at our motel by myself, thinking about all the things in my life that were going wrong. We spent the entire day together, and when it was time for me to go home, we started kissing in the car. I actually saw my wife in the backseat. I freaked out and yanked myself away.

"I've got to go," I said. "Oh, this is wrong."

I got out of there as quickly as I could. I continued to feel a pull toward the teacher. But when she wanted to meet me again, I knew it was no good, and I wouldn't agree. At the same time, I didn't know what I was feeling. Rebecca and I had been married for almost five years, and we'd been arguing more and more in the past year. When Rebecca called to talk, I didn't know what to say to her.

"Something's wrong," she said. "I feel something's up with you."

After much cajoling, I broke down and told her what had happened. Obviously, she flipped, and she planned to drive up to Green Bay. I didn't want to hurt Rebecca, but I also couldn't get clear on what I was feeling about the teacher. My selfishness knew no bounds. I found myself wondering if I'd gotten married too young. Maybe I hadn't sown enough wild oats. *What is my thing for the teacher telling me?* I wondered. *If I truly loved Rebecca, why did I end up kissing this other woman? Is there something here? I don't know.*

So I met with the teacher again. Even before anything more could happen, I realized there was nothing real between us. But try telling that to Rebecca. She was furious, and rightly so. As soon as she got to my motel, she started in on me.

"Did you go see her again?" she said.

"Yeah, I did."

"Why are you seeing her? I can't believe you."

"I don't know why. I don't know what I want. I don't even know if I want you. I think I'm going to get a divorce, and I think I'm just going to go to LA."

Yes, I was a model for the most astounding immaturity. All I wanted was to fly to LA and sit by the beach. That's how out of touch I was with my family and myself. Rebecca looked like I'd struck her. She started to cry.

"Terry, just don't leave me," she begged. "Just don't leave."

Instantly, it all became clear: Watching her cry reminded me of how far I'd fallen. *She's asking me not to go, so I have to stay,* I thought. *I can't do that to her and the kids. I just can't. I'm a good guy.* Well, maybe I wasn't acting like a good guy, but I knew I wanted to be one.

What finally shook me out of my crazy fantasy was that teacher, actually. I saw her visiting another player on my team. *Wow, okay, I almost gave up my whole life, and someone who really loves me, for this tramp.* That was a huge lesson for me. Now I'm sure everybody else could see it, but I'd been so naive up until then.

I felt so lucky that I'd woken up before I'd lost everything. I went to Rebecca.

"I'm a fool," I said. "I saw that chick with somebody else. I think I idealized her, and I don't even know why."

Maybe because I viewed my father as "the bad man" in my household growing up, I looked at my mother as holy. Whatever she said was right. All women were good. But, of course, there are some conniving women out there, and some conniving men, too. And when you idealize the wrong people, it can ripple out into everything else.

Again, I felt very lucky I got the chance to realize I was just being a young dummy before it was too late.

So, going into the next season, I put everything I had into camp, and I mean everything. I really gave it my all. I did great, and the coaches liked me, and finally, I felt good. I had my whole family up in Green Bay to watch the last game before the coaches decided which players they were going to cut. It had been such a long, dark time, and we were all ready to celebrate. After the game, I was on my way into the locker room when I heard my name spoken by "The Turk," the guy who cut people.

Ugh, no, are you kidding me? I thought. *I know I did really well.*

Not well enough, apparently. And I was so close, too. There are forty-five players on a team, but they can keep fifty-three. So when they're putting together the season roster, they go down to forty-five, and then back up to fifty-three. Well, I didn't make it through the final cut. I couldn't believe it. Sterling Sharpe, who was one of the star wide receivers on the team at the time, saw me packing up my stuff.

"I can't believe they cut you, brother," he said. "You were doing your thing."

I had given it my all, and it hadn't been enough. I was devastated. We still had no money. And now I was cut again, and there was nothing to do but drive back to Flint. But I couldn't bring myself to go home just yet. Rebecca and I had my parents drive Naomi and Azi down to Flint, while we stayed behind an extra day to recover and kind of get our bearings. The day before, we'd been picking out places to live. That's how confident I'd been. And now it was all over.

As Rebecca and I drove back to Flint, it was the quietest ride. We were both contemplating all we'd been through, and all of the drama, even just in our own relationship. I didn't know where my head was at, now that my NFL dream was over. I'd been in it for a little bit, but after what had happened with the Rams, and now this, it clearly wasn't working out. I was unemployed. I was broke. I began to think maybe this was my punishment from God for all the acting out with pornography, the teacher in Milwaukee, and every other dumb decision I'd made. *Do I go back to school? Do I get a job?* I was so exhausted, I couldn't think anymore.

"Let's just stop at a hotel, any hotel, and take a break," Rebecca said. "If we get some sleep, it will feel a little bit better."

Rebecca was always talking tremendous amounts of sense, but I never listened to her, except for in my rock-bottom moments. It was only when I was beat down that I could finally see the world as it was. Looking back, I don't know how she stuck it out with me through all of this. I can only imagine she saw me as the ego-driven, immature narcissist that I was, and realized I was responding and reacting without thinking, and so she figured she had to think for both of us until I grew up a little. It wouldn't surprise me to learn that she'd looked over at me sometimes and thought: *I can't leave you. You need me. You'll die without me because you're an idiot.* She was right, and I'm so lucky I had her then, and I'm so lucky I have her now.

Of course, where did we end up stopping? The place I most hated and swore I'd never go back to: Kalamazoo. But there we were. We checked in to a motel, and I went right to bed. I couldn't face reality anymore, and so I lay down and curled up in a ball. Rebecca sat next to me and put her hand on my back.

"I'm going to call your mother to find out how the kids are doing," she said.

This was before cell phones, so we hadn't talked to my parents since they'd left. As soon as Rebecca got on the phone with Trish, she handed it to me.

"Terry, I was praying for you to call," Trish said. "The San Diego Chargers have been calling here. And the Green Bay Packers called. They're trying to find out where you are, but they can't get ahold of you."

"What?" I said.

"Call your agent, now," she said. "Everybody is trying to get ahold of you."

As I hung up and dialed my agent, all I could think was: *Please, God, please.*

My agent had been trying to reach me all day, and I got him on the phone right away.

"The San Diego Chargers want you on a plane right now," he said. "They want you on the team this week, like as soon as you can get there. Go to the nearest airport, take everything you have, and put it on a ticket to go to San Diego."

Rebecca and I were jumping up and down on the bed.

It's not over, I thought. *It's not over.*

Just like with my college scholarship—and the NFL draft— just when it had seemed like everything had ended for me, my NFL dream was still alive.

We made a plan. Rebecca would go back to Flint to get the kids and drive out to meet me in San Diego. On the way, she dropped me off at the airport. I got a ticket and flew from Flint to Chicago, where I had to change planes. I had just boarded my flight from Chicago to San Diego, when I heard a commotion in the front of the plane. I looked up and these two burly security guards were headed my way.

"Is that him?"

"Yeah, that's him."

This can't be happening.

"You, you," the one guy said. "Come with us."

They pulled me off the plane in front of everybody.

I was terrified because the only thing I could think was that Rebecca had gotten in a car accident, or something horrible had happened.

No, God, please don't. Not such great news followed by the worst.

They had me standing on the Jetway.

"What's the nature of your business?" one guy said, his voice hostile.

"I'm going to San Diego for business."

They wouldn't tell me anything. Finally, I'd had enough.

"Sir, I'm going there to sign a contract with the San Diego Chargers," I said. "I just got cut from the Green Bay Packers. I'm a football player. That's what I do."

They looked at each other, and then they apologized and explained. At that time, anybody who was black and bought a ticket at a small-town airport with cash was dealing crack. So they'd thought I was a drug dealer. They looked embarrassed.

"Hey, can we get an autograph?" one guy asked.

Really? After that kind of nasty racial profiling, you want an autograph? But this was no time to be Mr. Militant. I was just so glad that everyone in my family was safe. AND I was going to the Chargers. "Yeah, cool," I said. "Just get me to San Diego."

My grandmother always said I missed my money on that one, but I was too happy to sue anyone just then.

I arrived in San Diego. After Green Bay, where everything had been heavy—my mood, the weather, the food, the relationship issues, getting cut at the last minute—it was paradise. There was the sea and the sun, and it was incredible. They put me in a hotel where all of the players were staying. I WAS ON THE TEAM. My first day was team picture day, and I didn't even know the other guys yet, but there I was, part of the team. I looked around and there was Junior Seau, and everyone else. They showed me to my locker, and at practice they threw me into play right away. I didn't even know the system yet, but I didn't care. I would learn it. After two seasons of being on the sidelines, I was more than ready to play and earn my way.

Meanwhile, Rebecca drove cross-country, by herself, with our two kids. I told her to go slowly and stop whenever she got tired, but she was determined. She was ready to get out of my parents' house and start a new life, and after everything that had happened, she really wanted all of us to be together again. I did, too. Four and a half days later, she arrived at the hotel and came into my room with the kids.

"Hey, babe, what's up?" I said. "How you doing?"

"Hey, honey, how are you?"

"Yeah, yeah, let's get the bags," I said. "Let's go, I've got to get to practice."

She fell onto the ground in a ball of tears and wept and wept.

"What's wrong? What's happening? This is a good time. We're doing well."

"I can't," she said. "I don't know what to do. I'm tired."

I hadn't realized the whirlwind of everything I'd put her through. All of the stress and the changes were just too much, and now that she'd made it to a safe place, she had to release everything she'd struggled so hard to keep inside.

"Babe, this is our new life," I said.

We just looked at each other, and it was so good. I'd made so many empty promises to her out of my sense of entitlement. I'd gotten us into so many problems with money. I'd kept saying things were going to get better, but they'd only gotten worse. And now, finally, we were in San Diego. I was on the team. Sometimes the change of scenery allowed us to see each other in a new way, and that was one of those moments. We were both so relieved and happy to be there.

We settled in and rented a little Ford Escort. We needed two cars, so I could go to practice and she could take the kids where they needed to go. I was at practice when I had a funny feeling I should take the Pathfinder home at lunch and drive the Escort back. When I pulled up at the stadium in the Escort, a man approached me.

"Terry Crews?" he said. "You have a Nissan Pathfinder? We're here to get it."

They'd finally caught up with me, but I'd managed to pull it out of the fire once again, and just in time. I was so relieved.

"It's not here," I said. "As soon as I get paid, I'll get you all of your money."

"Cool," the guy said. "Can we get an autograph?"

B Y THIS POINT, I WAS SO GLAD TO STILL BE IN THE GAME, and I had no more bubbles left to burst. I was fortunate because football was never my be-all and end-all, but I saw so many guys who got worn down under the realities and the physical brutality of the NFL. Some of that was really dark to witness, but as long as I was there, I was going to play my hardest and enjoy how far my perseverance had taken me.

In hindsight, I can see now how my double life created two distinct personalities in me: One was this big grandstanding, moralizing person who viewed life according to the Pollyanna principle. My optimism was eclipsed only by my drive to win at all costs, and I wasn't going to let anybody get in my way, not even my wife or other family members. I saw every criticism as a takedown and an attempt to stifle my greatness, and I morally harangued anyone who disagreed. Playing football kept me in a world of slogans and mantras: *"No pain, no gain." "Those who stay will be champions." "Winning is everything." "Work hard, play harder."*

But when I was alone, it was like all of that fake optimism caught up with me. My faults and failures were always right there to remind me that I wasn't practicing what I preached. Acting out with pornography created a spiral of depression that sent me right back to more acting out. Which in turn created more shame. So I felt the need to do something great and praiseworthy in order to prove to myself I wasn't as bad as I seemed. I'm sure I was hell to live with, and I am truly thankful to my wife and family for not giving up on me during this time in my life.

I can never forget the people who'd helped me and believed in me along the way, and while I was on the Chargers, I finally had the chance to acknowledge one of them. We had a game in Kansas City, and I wanted to fly Coach Lee in to see me play. I couldn't get him sideline passes, but I had tickets for him, and I figured what really mattered was for him to know how much I appreciated him. I called him up.

"I want you to come out here," I said. "And I want you to see what one good word to a little boy can do."

I'd told my Chargers coaches how much Coach Lee meant to me, and one of these coaches ended up meeting Coach Lee at the hotel bar and giving him sideline passes and coach's credentials. I can't even tell you how special that was for me: Here was Coach Lee, the first person who'd ever really believed in me, sitting there as a coach, on the side of an NFL game, watching me play. It was one of the happiest moments of my life. Seeing him there, it was so clear to me: *Dreams do come true. It takes a lot of work. But it can happen.* I was very aware that I owed so much of what I'd accomplished to Coach Lee, and I let him know it, too.

"Man, you have no idea," I said. "If you had not told me I could do it, I wouldn't be here."

This is one of the central facts of my life. There were just too many other negative words out there. But, thankfully, that one positive word from Coach Lee is the one I held on to, and I'm grateful to him to this day.

My debut season with the Chargers was just the rejuvenation my football career and my marriage needed. I was living my NFL dream, but I'd never lost sight of the fact that entertainment was still my first love. Darwin came out to visit me, and we drove up to LA. I'd met a really cool guy, Devon Shepard, who was a young staff writer on *The Fresh Prince of Bel-Air*. We went to NBC studios and attended a taping, which was amazing. Afterward, we were in the parking lot, and I got to meet Will Smith. He had this white Bronco, which was *the* car back then—this was before it became the OJ Bronco. And he had this customized DJ Jazzy Jeff and the Fresh Prince carpet in the back, and these huge speakers. He turned them all the way up, and they set off all of the alarms in the parking lot. I loved *The Fresh Prince of Bel-Air*. That was one of the best sitcoms ever, and I can still watch it to this day. Talking to Will, and having him be so cool to us, and make jokes, and just be so affable, was amazing. *That's how a star is supposed to be,* I thought.

Devon took us to Roscoe's Chicken and Waffles, and on the way, we passed by *The Arsenio Hall Show,* which was the hottest show just then. At the restaurant, people were coming out of the taping, and I could feel their excitement. We were right by Paramount Studios, and Devon was sharing with me all of these stories about what entertainment was like, and I was enthralled. I drove the whole two and a half hours back to San Diego with stars in my eyes. I still never saw myself as an actor, but I knew Hollywood was where I wanted to be eventually. First, though, I was all about making the most out of my time in the NFL.

CHAPTER 11

WHAT I'M WORTH

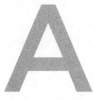ND THEN . . . YOU GUESSED IT. AFTER ONE year on the team, I got cut the last weekend of camp the following year. Now, this was the third team that had let me go in as many years. It was a tremendous blow, and it would have been impossible not to reassess my situation. Even Rebecca, who hadn't let me give up on so many occasions, was starting to have her doubts.

"You know, honey, maybe you're not that good," Rebecca said.

POW. I felt that. It hurt. Her criticism was honest, but to me, it was like she was personally trying to take me down. I had no strength left to fight. At the same time, that was one of those rock-bottom moments when I knew I had to acknowledge her good sense. *Maybe I'm not that good,* I thought. Now, that went right down to my core, the part of me that had done anything to keep the peace and make people like me. *I'm not worthy of the*

NFL. I'm worthless. I'm unlovable. That was my darkest fear, which I had fought so hard against my entire life, since I was a little kid waking up in a wet bed after a night of my father's drinking and my parents' violent fights.

But I wasn't a kid anymore. I was a grown man. I'd accomplished something in my life, and not just anything, either, but the realization of my NFL dream. I reassessed. *Wait a minute. My wife loves me. My kids love me. My parents love me. So that's not the issue. I'm not unlovable. I just need to be a better football player.* That was a discouraging thought, but it felt totally manageable. If I'd taken this latest rejection and decided it meant I was unlovable, that would have been a problem, because there was nothing I could do about that. But if I looked at it as a job that hadn't worked out, that was okay, because I could do something about that. Once I removed my emotions from the situation, I felt so much less discouraged. I made a plan. I would work harder. I would study my plays. I would convince the Chargers to give me another chance, or I would find another team that would.

Every week, the coaches called me.

"Terry, we're going to sign you next week. Just sit tight."

I viewed these phone calls as a sign that I was on the right track, so I stayed in San Diego, living on my own money. Someone else would have acknowledged that it wasn't working out, stopped the game, and moved on. But the codependent pleaser in me wouldn't let go.

Once again, we had no money coming in, and I had to figure out a way to get by. And then it hit me: I would draw on my other talent. I spent about three weeks on a portrait of Chargers player Ronnie Harmon on the field with the city of San Diego behind him. And then I went into the locker room. I was really nervous. I was very aware that I'd recently been a peer, and everyone knew I'd been cut, and I didn't want anyone's pity. On the other hand, I knew I was a good painter.

"Hey, guys, this is what I do," I said, holding up the painting. "If anyone here would like to have a painting of you, your kids, or anything else, I can do it for you."

It was a very humbling experience. I could definitely feel that everyone in the room was uncomfortable. But then, Ronnie stepped up and bought the painting I'd done of him, and that made me feel better about the whole situation. He also had us over for Thanksgiving dinner that year, which meant so much to me, especially after I'd experienced the feeling of becoming invisible after I'd been cut in the past.

I ended up doing paintings for four or five guys on the team. Each painting brought in about a month's income, which meant Rebecca and the kids and I could eat and live for that long off every painting I sold. And that's how we survived.

I developed a new Sunday afternoon routine while I was waiting to return to the team. As my teammates were playing, I went into my garage, turned on my radio, and painted for hours and hours. There were definitely moments when it was hard to hear the game going on without me but, lost in a painting, I could forget my pain. Time stopped. I was in the zone, as I'd sometimes been in sports, with everything going so well, and my awareness so heightened, it was almost as if time had slowed down, allowing me to achieve this perfect union with what I was doing.

It was difficult, though, because the Chargers went to the Super Bowl in Miami that year, and I knew I was supposed to be on that team. At the same time, I'd done a big painting of former Green Bay Packers player Bart Starr for the Fellowship of Christian Athletes, with whom he was active, and they flew Rebecca and me to the Super Bowl to present it to him. I kept bumping into my former teammates. It was awkward because people kept telling me that I should have been playing with them, and I wanted to be, but I was there because of my art instead.

I wasn't on the sidelines for long. I did a stint with the World Football League in Germany. Rebecca and the girls came over with me for that, but it was dismal. I was so grateful to be one of only seven players out of 300 to make it back to the NFL that year. And then the Washington Redskins signed me, so we moved across the country so I could begin playing for them—if I could make the team.

W HEN I ARRIVED AT REDSKINS CAMP, I MET THE TEAM'S linebacker Ken Harvey, who was not only one of the stars of the team, but also one of the first NFL linebackers to make big money. The coaches had us do a drill together. I hit him so hard that he started bleeding, and he still has a scar on his neck to this day.

Everybody looked at me like they couldn't figure out what I was doing, pummeling him like that. Well, as far as I was concerned, I had to make this team, and that was how I'd always done it: hit hard, make an impact, get noticed. My main ability in the NFL was to take tremendous amounts of pain. That was a valuable skill. When I could hit somebody and get up, the coaches told me I was winning.

Ken ended up taking a liking to me, this kid who'd been bounced around a lot and was desperate to make his team. Before camp was even over, he invited Rebecca and me over to his house for a barbecue. I assumed he was just being polite, and there'd be a huge crowd there. But when we arrived, it was just the four of us. He didn't know whether I was going to make the team or not, but he didn't care. He had a great heart. He'd scratched his way into football like me, as a walk-on to the team at a junior college, and he and his wife had been married about the same amount of time as Rebecca and me. So even though he lived in a huge mansion and had housekeepers, and Benzes, he was out there cooking for us on his grill, and telling really bad jokes, which was something else we had in common.

I ended up making the team and it felt so good! I felt like I'd showed Rebecca that I *was* good enough to be in the NFL, and somehow or someway, all of these coaches had had it in for me over the years. I always had an excuse to prove her faith in me was justified: "I am that good, but they just have to keep their superstar on" or "The general manager doesn't like me." The truth was, I had no idea why I was getting cut sometimes, while making the team other times, but I did a good job of finding reasons for when I did, and excuses for when I didn't.

I spent the next year being Ken's backup, and we became really good friends. On our nights off, he invited me to go shoot some pool, have some chicken wings, or just hang out and talk. He liked to write, and he admired my paintings, and so we bonded over art. These nights were such a relief after what I'd seen earlier in my NFL career, with the guns, and the drugs, and the strip clubs.

Ken and his wife were always taking Rebecca and me out to these fancy functions we couldn't otherwise afford. Because they never had to pay, they never let us pay, and they were just so nice about it. I still had my trusty old Pathfinder, and when it broke down, Ken let me borrow his Benz. Now, *that's* a friend.

Ken got hurt during a game, and I got to go in because I was his backup. For three consecutive plays, I made all three tackles.

He was on a gurney, on the sideline, and when he heard my name three times, he ran back into the game.

"What?" I said. "Just stay out."

"No, no, you've got to get out," he said. "I cost a couple million dollars. You cost a couple hundred thousand. Who are they going to keep if you're doing well?"

I used to always joke that the only obstacle to my NFL career was Ken Harvey, because if he'd just stayed out that game, I could have totally made it.

Ken was more than just a friend. He was my hero. He took me under his wing and became my big brother in many ways. In fact, going into my second season on the Redskins, I fired my agent in favor of his, which didn't end up being a good idea, but I wanted to do it because I admired Ken so much.

During contract negotiations, I was told I would be given a tender offer by the team, which was the minimum I should be paid based on my tenure in the NFL, according to the NFL Players Association. Only everyone told me not to sign the tender offer, even though that's what I was supposedly worth.

"Don't sign it," my coach said. "Because once the tender offer period is over, we can resign you for whatever we want."

"That doesn't make sense," I said. "Why are you giving it to me anyway?"

"Well, that's how it works," he said. "We're going to sign you for much less, and if you sign this now, it will count against the team's salary cap."

I didn't like being paid less than the NFL said I was worth. I wanted to earn the amount of the offer, which was a good amount of money. I went to my agent.

"This doesn't make any sense," I said. "If they can just sign me for whatever they want, then why are we even going through all of this?"

"Well, you can sign it, and they'd have to pay you that amount," he said.

"Well, why can't we do that?"

"Because they'll probably cut you."

"I'm tired of just fooling around," I said. "I need to really make some money now, and with my tenure, this is what the NFL says I should be paid."

"Okay, let's do it and see what happens."

So I went into the office to sign it. The defensive coordinator stopped me.

"Terry, don't do it," he said.

"Well, sir, this is what the NFL says I'm supposed to be getting paid," I said.

So he let me go. But even the secretary weighed in on the issue.

"Are you sure you want to do this?" she said.

"Yeah, this is the offer you're giving me."

So I signed it. Oh, boy. The next day, the team's GM sought me out.

"You shouldn't have done that, Terry."

"What? That's what the NFL says I should be getting paid, that's what I should be getting paid."

He gave me a look that said: *You're about to be getting paid nothing.*

We were still in training camp, and Ken pulled me aside at practice.

"Terry, they got it in for you, man," he said.

He was clearly right. When I went into the weight rooms, I was ignored. When I went into the meeting rooms, I was ignored. It was like being part of a cult, something I knew a thing or two about after my time in Maranatha.

Whoa, what happened? I wondered, trying to hang on.

We had these depth charts for the special-team players, and I went from number one to number six. Suddenly, there were people that nobody had ever seen or heard of who were over me, and let me tell you it wasn't because of anything I failed to do on the field. I tried to act like everything was normal. Clearly, it was not.

"Dude, they're going to cut you, man," Ken said. "I can feel it."

I was afraid he might be right. So I went to the NFL Players Association and spoke with their representative.

"How is this legal?" I said. "Like, what's going on?"

"Well, you're not a star, and basically, there's nothing we can really do."

That was my first and last experience with those NFL union guys.

I talked to Rebecca. I talked to my agent. We tried to figure out if there was anything I could do to turn things around. Well, if I had the choice between being re-signed for too little money or being cut and earning no money, I knew which way I'd go. So my agent went to the team and said I was willing to sign the second offer, even though it was the NFL minimum for my position and less than half of the deal I'd just signed. They re-signed me for less, and I breathed a huge sigh of relief. I immediately went up in the depth charts again. Disaster averted. But there was still one problem. Because I'd signed when I had, the additional money in my first contract had counted against their cap. I'd cost them money.

"Man, this is going to be ugly," Ken said. "I don't know what's gonna happen."

Actually, now that I'd accepted less money, everything was fine. In fact, it was really good. I had a great camp. My contract went through. There was a big barbecue with all of the coaches, and the players, and our families.

"Congratulations, Terry, you made it," my linebacker coach said to me.

It was wonderful. Everyone was kissing my kids. I mean it was great. I started making plans as soon as we were driving home. Rebecca and I always waited until the absolute last minute to sign leases and enroll our kids in school, because we never knew where we were going to be from year to year. Now we knew, at least for the next season. *I made it another year,* I thought. *What a relief.*

"Let's put the kids in school, Becky," I said. "We're good."

That day, she signed our lease and enrolled our kids for the school year.

The next day, I went to practice. I worked out. I did my thing. And then we all went to lunch. The quarterback, Gus Frerotte, gave me a confused look.

"What are you doing here?" he said. "Didn't you get cut today?"

"What are you talking about?" I asked.

"The newspaper says you got cut."

"No, I didn't. I'm here. Nobody told me."

"No, no, no, you got cut, man."

I went to the coach. He barely looked up from what he was doing.

"Coach, what is he talking about?" I asked. "Did I get cut?"

"Oh, no, no, don't believe the papers," he said. "The papers are ridiculous. They got that wrong. Look, let's just go to practice and continue to practice."

So I went to practice, worked as hard as I could, showered, and went home. I hadn't been home long when the phone rang. It was my coach.

"Terry, we need you to come back up here and bring your playbook."

"But I made the team."

"We're going to cut you."

All I could think was, *But yesterday, you were kissing our kids.*
Let me tell you, the NFL got me ready for the entertainment
industry because it does not get colder than that. This truly was
one of the central lessons I needed to learn in my life: *Never
make decisions based on money.* I'd been warned, and I should
have listened. Signing that contract was a mistake, pure and
simple. As I learned over time, if I'm doing my dream job, that's
enough, and once I become one of the top guys, the money will
come. I also got that I should never worry about minimums.
The truth about a minimum salary requirement is that if they
can pay you less, they will. Always. Instead of getting my ego
wrapped up in numbers and what they supposedly said about
my worth, I should have figured out ways to become more valuable, and never bothered myself over the other stuff. Had I increased my value to the organization, we never would have had
a "minimum pay" discussion again.

Rebecca and I ended up staying in the area for another year
because the kids were in school, and during that whole time,
Ken never deserted me. Even though he was on the team, he
was still my friend. He even gave me a little money here and
there when I needed it. His loyalty meant so much to me. And I
have to say that, overall, this was one of the first times Rebecca
and I maintained relationships and were still treated like insid-
ers, even though I was off the team. That camaraderie got me
through many dark days that year. Ken, especially, did everything he could to keep my spirits up. I really did not know what
I was going to do next.

"Hold on, man, it's going to be great," he always said. "It's
going to be good."

———

THAT SAME YEAR, THE EAGLES PICKED ME UP FOR THE playoffs. But I never played, and then they told me they weren't going to re-sign me. I was filler for the team during the playoff season, and I eventually learned I wasn't going to go to camp with them. Next, I worked out for the San Francisco 49ers. By that point, I'd been on six teams in seven years. I was running out of teams, and steam. Even more important, I could feel that something had changed for me.

During the workout, the coach threw the ball at me so hard it dislocated my finger. I was lethargic and cynical about all of the drills. I felt horrible. I went home to Herndon, Virginia, where we lived during my stint with the Redskins. I laid it out for Becky. "I don't think my heart's in this anymore," I said.

Rebecca gave me a long look.

"Remember when we met, and we were dating, and we got engaged, and you said, 'I'm going to play in the NFL, and then we're going to move to LA, and we're going to make movies,'" she said. "It's time to move to LA."

"Are you really serious? You think this is it?"

"Your heart's not in it. Let's go. We don't have anything here."

I knew she was right.

"You know what? Let's go. We've got nothing to lose."

My whole plan was to be behind the scenes. I'd never acted before, and that was not even a consideration for me. I was going to be an animator or special-effects artist, and, eventually, I was going to write, direct, and produce my own projects. In 1995, I'd even filmed a little movie I'd produced, *Young Boys, Inc.,* with my old NFL buddy Anthony. We'd gotten kicked out of locations in Detroit. We'd gotten beat down. We'd run out of money. We never even finished the movie. Still, it was one of the best times of my life.

During my time with the Redskins, I'd tried to generate heat for *Young Boys, Inc.,* even throwing a big fund-raiser partway through the season. As was my way back then, I spent nearly $20,000 on an event meant to impress my teammates, and I didn't earn a single cent on the whole endeavor. But now that we were going to LA, I could take the film with me and finally make something happen with it. I was an extreme dreamer.

The only thing I felt like I had still tying me to Virginia was Ken. We went out one night, and I told him I was moving to LA.

"Okay, do you know anybody?" he said.

"No."

"What are you going to do?"

"I don't know."

"So you're just going to up and leave?"

"Yeah, we're going to load up and get out of here."

"Man, you need anything?"

"Thank you, man."

He gave me a couple thousand dollars to help us move, and that was huge. During our transition, we spent about a month at my parents' house in Flint, during which time I arranged my official retirement from the NFL and got my severance. We moved to LA and landed in an itty-bitty extended-stay hotel in Burbank. We didn't know a soul. At the time, Naomi was ten and Azi was eight. Not long after we arrived in LA, Rebecca got pregnant. We were overjoyed, but I was also terrified.

That was an extremely stressful time. We didn't have any money, and I had too much pride to get a job. I'd come from the NFL, I'd made a film, and I was going to get into the business. I was sure that all counted for something. Well, I soon found out that Hollywood didn't give a damn. Again, Rebecca remained supportive.

"Look, whatever you have to do, do," she said. "But this is the thing. How long do you think it's going to take for you to realize if it's not going to work? Like how long will we be here? Is it three years, four years, what?"

"We are never leaving," I said. "Football is done. But this I can do forever. I will never be happy doing anything else."

It was the absolute truth. Somehow I knew: Hollywood was in my lifeblood.

"If we're ninety-nine years old, and we hit it big then, it will all be worth it," I said.

"Okay, got it," she said. "That was all I needed to know. We're going to be in California. Cool. I've got you. So let's do it."

Rebecca's faith in me never wavered, but now she was all about talking sense into my stubborn, lumpy head. We were broke, because I wasn't being smart.

"Terry, you need a job," she said. "We're running out of money, and you're doing the filmmaker thing, but you need to do the workman thing."

"But I can't do that," I said. "That would hurt my image."

I still thought having Hollywood see me as a former football player was going to help, but as I was learning again and again, Hollywood didn't care. I'd created a portfolio and put it in at Disney's hand-drawn animation department. People there were taking notice, but their method often was to give notes on applicants' work five or six times before deciding to hire them, and I didn't have that long. I went over to DreamWorks, and their animation department was creating *Prince of Egypt*. I did some hand drawing for them, and I got some notes on my portfolio, but again, it would have been a long time coming. Trying to make money as an artist in Hollywood just seemed too ridiculous.

During this time, Ken was my lifeline. He kept sending me gold coins from this gold bullion he had in his savings.

"Look, when you get into trouble, take the coin to a jeweler. Each coin is an ounce, and whatever the price of gold is per ounce that day, they'll give you."

Every couple of months, he sent me eight or ten coins. Looking back now, it seems like such a crazy way for me to have lived and supported my family for that long, but at the time I didn't feel like I had a choice. I had hocked Rebecca's ring, my watch. Whatever we had that I could sell, I had pawned.

Finally, I got ready to pawn our car. Rebecca stopped me at that.

"What are you doing?" she said.

"We've got to do this."

"No, we don't. You need a job. You need to just go to work."

"No, babe, it's going to work," I said.

That's what I'd always told her in college. It had worked then, but this was different. Our NFL dream was over, and we were about to have our third child.

"But if we lose the car, what are we going to do then?"

"I don't know, we'll find a way," I said. "I'll bike it. I don't care. We've got to do this to just get us by. We're only a minute away. We're almost there."

Of course, we were really far away, but I didn't know it then. This went on for about a year. I hocked the car at this place that gave us about $2,500 and let us continue to use it. We had to pay back the money at an exorbitant interest rate, and if we missed even one payment, they would come and take the car. Rebecca couldn't believe it. She threw up her hands at me and prayed:

Lord, please help this man, because he's being a fool and nobody can talk any sense into him!

We had nothing left. One day, I called Ken. "Ken, hey, dude, I need some help," I said. "You know, we've pawned everything. Can you just send me a little bit?"

"Terry, I can't do it."

In all of the years we'd been friends, it was the first time I'd ever heard him say no, ever. I was stunned, and I didn't know what to say.

"I can't do it," he said again.

He was really saying no. I didn't get it.

"Why?"

"Hey, man, I just, that's enough," he said. "I have officially given you all of the money I can. The reason I gave you the coins was because my wife would have felt uncomfortable with me writing checks, and so I was just trying to slip things to you like that, but it's not right. I can't give you any more money."

He had given me a lot of money over the years. But instead of being grateful, I got mad. *What is this?* I thought. But, of course, I knew I couldn't say that to him.

"That's all right," I said. "Hey, I understand. No problem. I'll talk to you later."

I hung up mad. And then it hit me: *Why are you angry with the only man who ever helped you? Why does it bother you so much that he told you no? You feel like he owes you, and he's the only one who's ever helped you. He doesn't owe you anything. You are a grown man. You are on your own. You need to do whatever it takes, and your wife has been telling you this the whole time, but you didn't listen to her.*

And then I had an epiphany that changed my life: *There's no looking cool. There's no being hip. There's no pro-football-player image. I need to start all over again, because no one is coming to save me. I've got to do it for myself, and I've got to do anything it takes.*

That was it for me. I knew what I had to do. I went to Rebecca.

"Ken's not doing it anymore," I said. "I've got to do it. I'm going to get a job."

"Yeah," she said, as in, *WHAT HAVE I BEEN TELLING YOU ALL ALONG?*

That week, I went to a place called Labor Ready in North Hollywood. Every morning, I showed up at five a.m., and they assigned me manual labor for the day, for which I was paid $8 an hour. For an eight-hour day, after taxes, I earned $50. It was basically a halfway house, because so many of the workers had just come out of prison. There were a lot of drug addicts. They were in really rough shape. On my first day, I looked at the people around me. They were itching, scratching and dirty, and they were there to sign up to earn their money, just like me.

The boss sent me to a place in the Valley called White Cap, and they handed me a broom. I had tears in my eyes when I started sweeping. I swept for eight hours.

I've got to do anything it takes. I've got to do anything it takes.

Some of the other workers came up to me.

"Hey, hey, hey, man," one of the guys said. "You look familiar."

It was clear he didn't really know who I was, but I didn't look like any of the other guys. I looked like a pro-football player. So he wanted to prove something.

"You don't know me, man," I said.

I was wearing a hat. I pulled it down and made myself keep quiet.

Just take it, I thought. *Understand it's on you. No one's going to help you. You might be sweeping floors for a while. This might be your life now.*

FALLING AWAKE

FAMILY

CHAPTER 12

ATTITUDE ADJUSTMENT

AYBE I DIDN'T WANT TO ADMIT IT AT THE TIME, but I needed that humbling. I needed to be broken. Because the moment when you're broken is the moment when you can see what's really happening. While I was sweeping, for hour after hour, I thought about how my wife kept telling me to do the right things, and how I ignored her and went my own way. I thought about my parents, and how I thought I was better than they were, and how I resented "factory work" and stuck my nose up at anyone who did it. Even with all of the problems my mother and father had experienced, they'd sacrificed so much to make sure I could live a better life, and they both loved me with all of their hearts. Then I thought about Ken, the man who had given me money and friendship and truly was the reason I was even able to move out to California in the first place. Here, he had a wife and kids, but he believed in me enough to take money from them and give it to me. It struck me how good his family had been to me, and how wrong it had been for me to expect him to be responsible for me. I felt ashamed. When I got home from work, I called Ken.

"Man, I'm sorry," I said. "I was mad at you, and I had no reason to be."

"It's cool, man," he said. "I just want to see you make it."

"Thank you," I said.

That job was a breakthrough for me. Before that, I'd been so concerned about my ego, and how I looked, and how people saw me. My main concern was preserving my image, no matter what. Rebecca had constantly been on me to put our family first, but I was just too immature and self-centered.

When I was in the NFL, I felt so entitled because I played football, and I thought everyone should feel lucky to help me get what I wanted. If I didn't get what I wanted, I was resentful—and, honestly, mean—even to my own wife and kids. Well, let me tell you, that's not how the world works. And there's nothing like eight hours with a broom to set a man straight. After that, I knew I was willing to do anything for my family, especially now that we had another baby on the way.

Luckily, I only had to work as a janitor for about a week, and that week felt like a year. I'd had my humble time, and I knew I couldn't do that job forever. I got myself over to a temp agency as quickly as I could and passed their typing test. They put me at the Veterans Administration Hospital in North Hills, in a mobile office, filing papers that had been displaced by the Northridge earthquake. It was definitely a step up from janitorial work. But it was still a far cry from the NFL and my plan to finish my movie and put it out into the world as a way to gain entrée into the entertainment industry. On top of that, I earned $8 an hour, for eight hours of work a day, even though I would have gladly taken on extra hours to earn more. I'd humbled my-self, and we were still just barely getting by. I was soon depressed and wondering what had become of my life.

I didn't want to abandon my Hollywood dream, no matter what, so I stayed up all night watching movies as research for my film. I lived on hamburgers and fast food, and I stopped working out. I quickly gained thirty pounds, and let me tell you, it was not muscle mass. I was really out of shape. Even though I'd always cared about looking sharp, I started just throwing on a big T-shirt and some sweats, lumping around and creating the outward representation of how bad I felt inside.

My friend Mark, who I'd met during my time with the Chargers, tried to rescue me from the brink. He owned a beau-tiful house near San Diego, and when we were really struggling, he always told me that if I had enough gas in our car to get us down to see him, he'd take care of the rest. I had not missed a payment on our hocked car, and we'd been able to get it back, but we were *broke*. His place was paradise. The whole family swam in his pool. He barbecued and made us the most beautiful food. He even put gas in our car for the return trip. He was a true friend to me in my time of need.

Mark could see I was in serious decline, and he called me about it one day.

"Terry, are you working out, man?" he said. "Are you doing anything?"

"Nah, I'm done with that," I said. "I've been concentrating on this film stuff."

"Come on, you've got to work out," he said. "You can't let that body go to waste. You've been playing, you've got your NFL body, man, don't lose it."

"Yeah, yeah," I said, just to get him off the phone.

I was so depressed that, without being conscious of it, I'd

created a net-negative vortex, and I couldn't bring myself to work out. I knew I should, but I couldn't do it. Without anything to rouse myself out of my funk, I avoided taking care of myself, and I sunk lower and lower, while denying it was happening.

I think many men are like this. We don't acknowledge any negative changes in our appearance, and we continue to see ourselves as we looked at our best. I definitely deluded myself about my own weight gain until Rebecca came up behind me in the bathroom. And pinched my back fat. It was like she had slapped me awake.

"What did you do?" I said, tensing.

"It's cute," she said. "You're just so cute."

She did it again.

"Stop, stop, stop," I said.

It was as if the world had screeched to a halt. But I was still in denial.

"What are you doing?" I said.

"You got a little thing here," she said. "It's all right, honey. I love you. It doesn't matter to me."

Even with the burgers, and the sweatpants, and the weight I'd gained, I'd never acknowledged what was happening. I honestly never had. Suddenly, I looked in our bathroom mirror and saw myself as I truly was at that moment. I looked as miserable as I felt. I had dark circles under my eyes. My skin was broken out. *I'm tired. I'm out of shape. I look terrible. Something's got to change. I'VE got to change. I cannot go on like this anymore.*

Our pastor at our church in San Diego had once said something that had really stuck with me: If you do something for twenty-one days, it will become a habit, and that means you can change your life in twenty-one days.

Even though we were broke, I knew I couldn't use that as an excuse.

"Becky, I've got to take a little bit of money, and I've got to join a gym," I said. "Tomorrow."

"Okay, I've got no problem with that," she said. "You go ahead and do what you've got to do."

Now here was my next big shock. Not only did I have to pay to work out for the first time in my life, but also there was no schedule that told me what exercises to do and when to do them. I had to do it by myself, and I had to do it for myself. I didn't even know where to start. I just knew I had to get in my twenty-one days.

On that first day, as I walked around, it all came crashing down on me. I was a professional athlete. No, I wasn't, not anymore. Now I worked at the Veterans Administration, and I wasn't even in good shape. I was at least forty pounds overweight, with a spare tire of fat around my middle. I sighed and climbed onto a little recumbent bike. I got so depressed, I lasted only five minutes.

"I've got to go home," I said. "I can't do this."

I ran right out of there. But at least I'd gone. That was day one.

I went back the next day, stayed for maybe fifteen minutes, and then I went home. No matter how bad it felt, or how down I got, I made myself go back every day. By the twenty-first day, amazingly, I was actually doing a full workout.

Even more than that, three weeks was long enough for me to see a change. Honestly, my body hadn't really changed much in that time, but my mood had. I felt so much better, happier, and most of all, clearer. I realized there had been something wrong with my brain before because of my inactivity. It was almost as if my thoughts had become cloudy, and my spirit had become depressed. Now, by contrast, I felt so much better. There seemed to be something healing about the movement itself. I realized that some of my happiest days, ever, had been when I was running in the sunshine across a grassy football field. And then I came to understand that, as humans, we're meant to be much more active than we are. There was also something so positive about actually having an impact on my situation.

Let me tell you, I was hooked. I started eating right, the pounds came off, and that twenty-one days turned into years. Even though I was still right where I'd been, filing paperwork for eight hours a day, I noticed that everything else had changed for me. My mood was better, as well as my thinking, and my reactions to the things that happened to me, even when they weren't good in and of themselves.

That's why I always tell people to treat working out like the spa, not as something we force ourselves to do, but as an indulgence, a treat, an activity we do to get our minds together. Honestly, for me, it's really not about my body anymore. Working out calms me. And it's always been like that for me. When I was a little kid, I dealt with feeling scared or out of control by lifting the furniture. Now exercising is something I look forward to doing every day. I go to the gym to find my peace, especially now that I've got an iPod. That changed everything for me. I fill it up with my audiobooks, teaching tapes, books on anything I want to learn about—Hollywood, acting, writing, working out—not to mention great podcasts, amazing tapes by inspirational pastors, and music. Once I have all of that good stuff going into my system for an hour or two every morning, I feel good. I feel pumped for the day. It's honestly become my joy. This is why I always tell people it's the wrong approach to feel like we need to go to the gym to get in shape. Rather, we should adopt the attitude that because we're in shape, we must go to the gym.

WAS SOON LOOKING AND FEELING BETTER, BUT IT WAS still a very intense time. Rebecca was pregnant with our third child, and money was very tight. One night, I had a dream. I was at a high school football game, watching my son play on the field. I couldn't see his face because he was wearing a helmet, but I knew he was my son, and all of the other parents were complimenting me about how athletic he was. Only I didn't really care about his performance because I was so elated to have a son. In fact, when I woke up, I was disappointed to find I'd only been dreaming.

"Rebecca, I dreamt we had a son, and he was playing football," I said.

"That reminds me of a vision I had that I was in a big, beautiful house, standing on a large staircase, holding a baby boy," she said.

I put my hand on Rebecca's big belly, convinced there was a boy in there.

"It's a boy," I said, giddy with excitement.

"No, Terry," she said. "I'm telling you, it's a girl."

Rebecca knew the baby was a girl and told me so whenever I brought up the possibility that she was pregnant with a boy. When the doctor was finally able to tell us the baby's gender, I was excited to find out for sure. Even once it was confirmed that Tera was indeed a girl, I still felt like she was my namesake. I'd always believed children should have their own name and was never interested in having a junior, but now I couldn't stop thinking about it. We saw a Terah in the Bible, and every time

Rebecca drove me to work at the Veterans Administration, we passed the Terra Bella exit on the 5 Freeway. Our third daughter's name would be Tera.

We were really struggling financially, but I did my best to hold on to my newly discovered positive attitude. When my alarm went off in the morning, before I could be crushed beneath the weight of the day's many stresses, I took a moment to think: *I'm alive. I'm alive. I can keep going as long as I'm alive.*

As I got dressed, packed my sack lunch with a sandwich and a PowerBar, and headed off to my eight hours of filing, I kept talking to myself the whole time: *I'm bigger than this. I am not this situation. This is not for me.*

For once, my confidence didn't come from an egotistical place. I really didn't agree with my circumstances. I knew I had greater value than $8 an hour. And I truly believe it was my ability to hold on to my sense of my own value that helped me to get through that time, even when things got worse. Our landlady went crazy and evicted us from our apartment, which we could barely afford. In order to keep the older kids in the same school, we took on an apartment across the street. It was a beautiful, barnlike structure, but small and more expensive. It seemed impossible that things could get any worse, or more stressful, but through it all, I hung on to my positive attitude. And I learned a major lesson, which is this: We determine our core value. We do. And we have to keep that value strong, no matter what.

Eating healthy, exercising, and working hard, even at a job I didn't love, all helped to keep my core value intact. But I still had bad habits that did not. We were able to afford an early iMac around this time, and soon I discovered that pornography was readily available on the Internet. These were the days of dial-up, and it took half an hour to load an image, but now there was no more sneaking out to video or liquor stores to get a fix. It was right at home and easily viewed with the push of a button. As the years went on, pornography became easier and easier to find and moved from pictures to full-on videos. It was like discovering I could jimmy the cable box all over again. I was able to become even more secretive, because my vice was pretty much evidence-free. Delete the image and search history and no one would be the wiser. But there was still a cost. My core value was continually battered by the pornography I snuck during times of stress. I couldn't objectify women like that, and keep a secret from my wife, and still feel good about myself.

During that time, my brother was in a terrible car accident. When the paramedics first arrived at the scene, his face was completely crushed, and they thought he was dead. He was airlifted to the hospital. They put metal plates in his face, and he had a very slow and painful recovery. I was devastated because I couldn't afford to fly home to visit him in the hospital, or to help him in any way. I felt so guilty, like this had happened to him because I hadn't taken good enough care of him. Here I was, out in LA, chasing my dream, when I should have been doing more for him. But I also knew I had my own family now, and I had to put them first.

It was a very difficult time, with so many emotions ricocheting around inside of me. *Is this ever going to work? Am I ever going to see anything out of this? What if I end up going back to Michigan anyway?* I knew that couldn't happen, ever, and I pulled myself together. I vowed, again, I'd never leave LA. And I limited my contact with my family back in Michigan, because talking to them made me feel like a loser.

I had made some initial progress with my film, *Young Boys, Inc.* I'd managed to attract the interest of director Reginald Hudlin, and my friend Anthony and I had found a manager.

But after nearly a year of being convinced it was about to happen for us at any moment, while Anthony lived on our couch, Anthony and I had a falling-out. That was it, not only with our friendship, but also with the movie. Clearly, it wasn't working out.

I still worked at the Veterans Administration, and I was also doing some bouncing at Timmy Nolan's Tavern and Grill in Toluca Lake. While there, I made a good friend, Trevor Ziemba, a police officer who also did security for fitness icon Billy Blanks. Trevor took a liking to me and used his influence to land me a job as a security guard on movie sets. This was the best thing to happen to me since I'd left the NFL. The job was a minimum of twelve hours a day, and it paid $12 an hour, $18 if we did music videos or commercials, so I instantly doubled my earnings.

There was just one problem: my attitude. Many of my co-workers had recently been released from prison. My supervisors had barely finished high school, and yet they talked to me like I was an ex-con: "Go over there. Tuck in your shirt."

I didn't like it. At all. In fact, I was often really offended. My ego once again reared its ugly head. Even though I was making good money, because I hated being talked down to, I became depressed. Even after the humbling of janitorial work, I felt I was still this big-time ballplayer, and now I was working for people beneath me. I was hurt by my situation, and so I had a very bad attitude.

And then, one day, it hit me: *Terry, look at what you have here. Really sit down and examine it.* I was working on my first movie, *Man on the Moon,* directed by Milos Forman and starring Jim Carrey as Andy Kaufman. There I was, at the Ambassador Hotel in downtown LA, wide-eyed, watching them move the lights and cameras, learning where the trailers were and what time they went to lunch. All I had to do for my job was to keep an eye on the extras, and so I had plenty of opportunity to observe everything else.

It was heaven. For lunch, there was steak and lobster and crab. I couldn't believe it. Now, of course, I've never had that again, even as an actor. But it was an amazing moment in my life. I'd literally been starving, you know, digging in the couch cushions in search of money for a burger. But now I could eat on the set, leaving Rebecca and the kids to have whatever was at home. And I was learning all of these film facts I never would have known unless I was on a set.

You are making more than double what you were making at your Veterans Administration job. They feed you. You get to spend twelve hours a day on a movie set, watching how all of these movies are made. This is basically paid film school, if you just open your eyes and see where you are.

I went home that night and told Rebecca what I'd realized.

"This is a godsend," I said. "My attitude has been totally wrong. Right now, I have to treat this job as if I'm getting paid a million dollars a day."

From that moment on, I ironed my shirts every day. I made sure my flashlight had batteries. I gassed up my car the night before. I decided everything was going to be a learning experience, and I was going to make good use of every single moment of every single day. I was the super security guard. There were days when I worked twelve hours, and I didn't have time to work out. So if I was at my guard post watching a trailer, and there was nobody in sight, I jogged in place for an hour, and that was my day's workout. I did push-ups. If there was a light post, I did pull-ups.

I wasn't going to let my brain atrophy, either, so I went to the library and filled up a gym bag with books on the entertainment industry. And when no one was looking, I sat and read book after book.

It had taken me only a few weeks to realize that standing there for twelve hours a day, staring at a wall, was making my brain shrink. Every hour was one in which I could learn. I had to constantly grow, and I'm still like that. My kids know that my car runs on gas and audio books. The way I look at it is that in the hour it took me to get from here to there, I could have learned something that changed my life. I was actually feeling positive about my job, and my life, for the first time in months. And then, one day, I was sitting down on a chair I'd found, when my supervisor came by.

"What are you doing sitting down?" he said.

"We can't sit down?" I said. "I'm doing my job."

"No, no, no, there's no sitting down on your post," he said.

"Oh, okay," I said, standing up.

Meanwhile, across the street, one of his friends who also worked for us, and was wearing the same uniform as me, was sitting in a chair.

"He's sitting there," I said, pointing across the way.

"No, no, no, I'm talking to you," my supervisor said.

So I folded up my chair, and I stood for the rest of the day.

Another day, that same supervisor came up and nodded at me.

"Go get some lunch," he said.

I nodded back and walked off to get lunch. Another supervisor saw me.

"Why'd you leave your post?" he asked.

"Well, I was told I could get lunch."

"No, you never leave your post."

So I went back to my post, and I wondered what was going

on. *Was this a game, or a mere unfortunate coincidence? Was I being hazed like I had been in football camp, or did these supervisors never talk to one another about how things were done?* The one thing I did know was that I never wanted anyone to ever have to discipline me. I wanted and needed that job too much. I decided I was going to do them one better. I threw away the chair, and I never sat again. I packed my own lunch along with my library books. I didn't care what anybody else was doing. I vowed they would never have to correct me, ever again. When my supervisor saw me jogging in place, he couldn't say anything about that.

"I'm up," I said, smiling.

"Go get some lunch," he said.

"I'm good," I said. "Don't worry about it."

I had my lunch in my bag, but I didn't want them to see me eat.

This was the best job I'd had in several years. Forget saving, but at least now we were at even, and we could eat and put gas in our car. On payday, I could never risk the extra time it took to have my check mailed to our house, so I always went into the security office to pick it up. There was one guy who loved to taunt me.

"You used to play in the NFL, right?"

"Yeah."

"Well, I mean, what happened? Why are you doing this?"

"Hey, man, everybody's got to work, right?"

I reached for my check. He pulled it back.

"Was it drugs? Were you on drugs?"

"No, sir, I was never on drugs."

"Oh, okay, so you just kind of messed up. It don't make no sense, man."

I kept my eyes on my check the whole time.

"Yeah, so what is it like in the NFL?" he said, holding the check.

I didn't want to answer, and I'd honestly become quite annoyed with all of the questions. But, looking back, if I was in his position, I'm sure I would have wondered the same thing. To say his interest was awkward was an understatement, but I was working, and for the moment, I had to avoid taking offense.

"Yeah, you know, it was tough," I said. "It was the NFL. May I have my check, please?"

"Yeah, here you go," he said, finally handing it over.

I knew this was the best job for me at the moment, and I had to hang on to it.

One day, I was standing at my post, with a book open, when my supervisor drove by and saw me. "Hey, hey, hey," he said. "Whatcha doing, reading?"

"Hey, man, now I understand," I said, closing the book and looking at him straight on. "I would never do this if there were people around, but I'm watching the area. And if someone comes by, the book goes down. But when nobody is here, I'm picking up a book. My brain is not going to just fry. I'm sorry. If that's wrong, then I've got to go. You've got to fire me."

Well, he looked at me, and it was a showdown. He didn't say anything.

"Dude, if you're going to stop me from reading, go ahead and fire me," I said.

He looked at me, and he looked at me, and it was a full-on game of chicken.

"No, man, go ahead," he said. "Go ahead."

Whew. I opened my book back up, and nobody ever said anything to me about my reading again. I even wrote scripts standing up sometimes, too.

During the months I did security on various film sets and

locations, multiple people from the different productions kept saying the same thing to me: "You really need to try acting. You've got a great look."

"Ugh, thanks," I said, but I had no intention of acting. I was an artist. I was going to work behind the camera. That's where I belonged.

Sometimes people could be pretty convincing, though. I was working on *End of Days,* starring Arnold Schwarzenegger, when his makeup artist approached me.

"What are you doing on this security detail?" he said. "You need to be in front of the camera."

"Okay, sir, thank you very much," I said. "That's cool."

But I couldn't think about acting. I was all about holding on to the job I had.

CHAPTER 13

KING OF THE MOUNTAIN

WORKED EVERY DAY I POSSIBLY COULD FOR ABOUT A year and a half. Producers had started requesting me because I was in shape, and I was ironed up, and so I was always busy. And then, finally, I had a rare day off.

My friend Trevor had called the day before, but I was tired when I got up in the morning, and I figured I'd call him back later. Rebecca had heard his message on the home phone, and she suggested I call him. When I did, he was freaking out.

"Yo, Terry," he said. "I was praying for you to call me. And you called me. Dude, get down to Venice Beach. Billy Blanks is down here. I'm down here."

"Whoa, whoa, what's going on?"

"They're doing these tryouts for this thing," he said. "You've got to come down. Dude, I promise you, you've got to come down here."

When I arrived at Venice Beach, there were 300 guys, running, jumping, doing obstacle courses, as part of the tryouts for this new show, *Battle Dome.* I found Trevor, along with Billy Blanks, and the show's producer, Stephen Brown.

"Okay, we're going to run you through different courses," Stephen said.

Well, I usually worked out first thing in the morning, but for some reason, I hadn't that morning. This meant I was fresh, and my muscles weren't tired at all.

I was up against all of these guys on Venice Beach. We were climbing ropes, doing the forty-yard dash. I beat everybody. Trevor kept pointing me out, and how well I was doing, to make sure the producers took notice. Then they put me in a wrestling match. I picked my opponent right up and slammed him right down.

"Dude, this guy," Stephen said.

They had *Access Hollywood* film some footage of me.

Well, I killed it. Everything they asked me to do, I did it almost two times better than all of the other guys. I drove home feeling lit up with how good I'd done.

"Becky, I don't know what that was," I said. "I don't know if they'll ever call me or anything, but let me tell you something, it was stupendous. What a day."

I was sure the producers were going to call me. A week went by. Two weeks. And then months went by, and I was back to my routine, doing security and reading and writing my scripts standing up. I was working on a movie called *Next Friday,* and they had me standing outside producer Matt Alvarez's trailer, right by Ice Cube's trailer.

As soon as I got home and walked through the door that night, Rebecca was flipping out. We didn't have a cell phone, so she'd been waiting for me to get home.

"*Battle Dome,* they called," she said. "They want to see you again."

When I phoned the producers for the details of the callback, I had a question.

"What do you want me to do?" I asked.

"Just be as wild and as charismatic as you can," the producer said.

So on the day of the callback, I went down to Cinema Secrets in Burbank and I had them paint my face in a pattern like Darth Maul. And then I went to a costume store, and I got a space age–looking leather belt, which I wore with spandex compression pants and boots. I looked absolutely ridiculous, like a total fool. But I was so hungry I was willing to do whatever it took. When I drove up to the Sony lot, the security guard took one look at my face and cracked up.

"Come on, dude, this is a movie studio," I said. "You can't act like you ain't seen nothing like this before."

"Aw," he said, still laughing as he gave me a pass.

When I walked into the audition waiting room, it was full of all of these huge meatheads who were also there to prove they had what it took to earn their big TV break. They all looked up at me and started laughing, all of them.

"Ah, look at him," one guy said, laughing and pointing at me.

I didn't know any of them, and I didn't care what they thought. I found a seat and went into my own zone. *I don't care, you can laugh all you want, I'm giving it all I've got, and when we go home at the end of the day, we'll see who's laughing then.*

Finally, my name was called, and I did my lines as big and boisterously as I could. They paired me up with two different people, and again, I went BIG. And then that was it. "Okay, thank you, Terry," the producer said.

As I drove home, I was at peace. I'd given it everything I had, and I felt good.

Several months passed by, and I was back to doing security and wondering if anything would ever come of my audition or my Hollywood dreams.

And then, one Sunday after church, the phone rang. It was a lady from Sony, telling me that they wanted me to go in and meet with them the next day. I was so excited I could hardly sleep. By the time I got to the production office, I was really nervous. I had no idea what this meant. I was ushered into a room with several guys, including Stephen Brown.

"Terry, you are one of our new warriors on *Battle Dome,*" he said.

"I'm on the show?" I said. "I'm on the show."

"You're in."

There was a moment where I didn't know what to feel, and I was just hollow. The ground went out from under me, and the sky lifted up, and I was just floating. I had been struggling so hard for so long, and then, just like that, everything changed.

I'm on a TV show. I'm an actor. I never even saw that as a possibility. But I am.

We got picked up for twenty-two episodes, and we would be shooting for six weeks. My character was named T-Money, and he was one of the bad guys, this gangster from Detroit who listened to rap music. I was so excited. And then, just like with my college scholarship and the NFL, I got a reality check. They wanted us to start working out with their trainers right away. Which was great, except for the fact that we weren't getting paid, and I'd already given my notice at the security firm. So I had to go back and take on more security shifts until we started shooting for real.

And then I was not at all prepared for how dangerous it was. It wasn't the other contestants I was worried about; it was getting my foot caught in one of the conveyor belts or other contraptions on the set. When we shot the first show, one of the games was basically King of the Mountain, except played on this cone that spun. So they put me on this thing, and I was battling this guy until I flew off. The next guy climbed up to fight the warrior on top. When he got thrown off, his foot turned all the way around so that it was facing the wrong way. From that day on, we were sending people to the hospital nonstop.

Luckily, I didn't go to the hospital. In fact, I became the show's breakout star. To make the situation even sweeter, the security force in charge of the show was my old company. Of course, I was experiencing fame only on a small level, but that was still the best possible turn of events I could have imagined.

"Hey, Terry, remember me?" my old supervisor said. "This is great, man. You're doing good."

"Hey, man, hey," I said.

Truth be told, the old me would have been tempted to pull rank and refuse to let them guard me. But I realized I didn't have to be rude to them. I didn't have to think that way anymore. I'd gotten out. I was in a different place.

But I still had a few obstacles along the way, like the Christmas from Hell. Shortly after I started on *Battle Dome* in 1999, we finally had enough money to fly back to Flint for Christmas. While we were there, Rebecca and I were invited to Detroit to have dinner with her longtime best friend. So we left the girls and little baby Tera with Big Terry and Trish. Now, I knew my father had relapsed in recent years, and so before we ever flew to Flint, I'd called him and given him a warning.

"I do not want my kids to experience you drinking, and to experience what I did when I was a kid," I said.

He'd agreed to be cool, and I'd decided to trust him.

Well, we were about to sit down to dinner when the phone

rang and Rebecca answered it. I could tell from her face that it wasn't good news.

"Big Terry is going crazy," Rebecca said. "Something is happening."

I got on the phone with my brother's wife.

"We're taking the kids to your aunt's house," she said. "Big Terry is hitting your mother. The kids are here. They're petrified. They don't know what to do."

"Oh, no, I told him," I said. "I told him."

My kids had never seen anything like that. I still had vivid memories of how awful and powerless I'd felt when I'd witnessed such violence in my home, and so I'd been determined they never would. The fact that Big Terry had done this in front of my kids seemed so disrespectful to me. Now I had to get that image out of their heads, because otherwise they would be shaken up forever. I definitely had been.

I dropped my wife off at my Aunt Paulette's house, and I called my brother. We met at our childhood home. When we walked in, it was horrible. I mean horrible. I can't even describe how awful it was. Big Terry had hit my mother so hard that her tooth was knocked sideways. Trish was crying. The air itself inside the house felt different. This was supposed to be the holidays, but it was manic.

"Trish, get in the car and go over to Paulette's house," I said.

As soon as she left, Marcelle and I turned on Big Terry as one. It all came back, all of the years when we had listened from our beds to the rumbling in the living room, the many times we'd cowered in the doorway while Big Terry hit our mother until she cried, the many times I'd felt small and powerless and scared.

"We're grown," I said. "You will never lay your hands on my mother again."

I punched Big Terry right in the face. I did. And then Marcelle punched him. All of those years of pent-up anger and grief came pouring out, and we beat him.

"Please stop," Big Terry begged. "Please stop."

I was crying, and punching him, and choking my words out through my tears.

"Oh, now you're going to cry," I said. "Now you're going to ask for help. I can't believe you, you big old man, you're running around here having everybody afraid of you for all of those years, and now you're afraid."

Marcelle was letting it all out, too. We wailed on Big Terry, slamming him around that house, until Big Terry finally fell to the ground.

"Please stop," Big Terry cried, standing up.

"Man, I'm not a little boy anymore," I said, knocking him back down. "And I can protect my mother now."

This went on for hours. Finally, our fight went all the way up to his bedroom, and he was just cowering there in the corner. All of a sudden, I couldn't do it anymore. I had thought I would feel like he was finally getting what he deserved and it would make me feel better. But I didn't feel better. I felt worse, because now I was a part of it, too. Now my mother was beat, he was beat, and this was my family at the holidays. It was just so horrible. I fell down onto my knees, and I cried. One good thing did come out of that mess, which was that he never touched my mother again. He realized we weren't playing, which is how I think it goes with a bully. But there was nothing we could do to save that holiday. We all tried to put on a happy face, but I think we were shell-shocked. My mother's tooth was sideways. We stayed our few days, and then we flew back home. It would be a lie to say I wasn't glad to go.

———

EXACTLY TWO YEARS AFTER WE MOVED TO LA, I GOT MY first real acting opportunity. The comedy of it is that if we hadn't been starving, I would never have tried acting at all. That's why I always say our struggle makes us who we are. If I'd had a comfortable job, and I'd been feeding my family without any problem, I would have kept pursuing my original dream of being an animator or a filmmaker.

But after *Battle Dome* aired, I was given the chance to audition for my first movie. I met with the casting director, Judith Holstra, for what I thought was a quick one- or two-day part in a movie. I got the part, and the next thing I knew, I was in Vancouver, with a major role in the latest Arnold Schwarzenegger movie, *The 6th Day*. My first day on set, a man approached me. It was Arnold's personal makeup man, Jeff Dawn.

"You look familiar," he said.

"You told me a year ago that I should be acting," I said.

"Oh my God." He laughed. "I'm making people rich here."

Well, I wasn't rich yet. Far from it. I'd just started acting, and I was scared I'd lose the part I'd been given. The production was shooting in Vancouver for four months. I didn't need to be there the whole time, but I was determined to stay.

"Hey, Terry, you're off for the next three weeks," one of the producers said. "We're going to send you back to LA."

"No, no, I'm just going to stay here," I said.

I was afraid if I left for even one day, they'd realize I was no good and fire me. Looking back, of course, that seems crazy to me. But I can understand now that this was my mind-set in the aftermath of the shakeup I'd experienced in the NFL. Because I was always getting cut, I was really insecure. I hadn't had a stable job since I'd left college, and so I assumed things weren't going to be any different now. I figured if I didn't leave, then they couldn't get rid of me, and they'd have to keep me around.

The problem was that I was far from home, all alone, and under tremendous pressure. I had no idea what I was doing as an actor, but I couldn't afford to lose the job, not only because we needed the money, but also because this was my Hollywood dream, finally coming true, and I was determined that I wasn't going to do anything to mess it up. And so I acted out, as I'd been doing when I was under stress since I was ten years old. But because this was the worst anxiety I'd ever experienced, I acted out in the most extreme way I ever had. I didn't sleep with another woman, but what happened was just as bad, perhaps even sleazier. It was like my porn addiction had stepped out of a magazine and come to life.

As soon as it was over, I regretted it immediately, just like I had with losing my virginity in college. I couldn't believe I'd actually let it go that far. *How did this happen? How did this happen? How did this happen?*

As I paced my hotel room all the rest of that day, I made a decision: There was no way I could ever tell Rebecca what had happened because she would definitely leave me. And so I would have to take my secret to my grave.

That was a dark time, and it got darker. Although acting out had alleviated my stress in the moment, it did nothing to help me in the long term, and my guilt and shame only made me feel more terrible. I was still lonely, and homesick, and worried I'd get fired at any moment. Only now it was worse because a part of me was also afraid to go home and face Rebecca with my secret inside of me.

Luckily I had one means of actually feeling better, even when I was at my lowest and loneliest. I started working out with a new trainer named Mike Talic, who ended up completely revolutionizing my approach to fitness. I never would have guessed the important role he was going to play when I met him. He was this rotund Slavic man, a former Olympic coach, and a sweetheart. He was not a pusher at all. On our first day at the gym, he stopped me before I could lift a single weight.

"Terry, Terry, let me show you what to do," he said in his thick accent. "Let me show you how to do it. You have to start with the basics."

I looked at him doubtfully.

"I've been working out all my life," I said.

"No, no, no, no, you do this move," he said, showing me. "Then you do that move. You keep doing it, it make you stronger."

I still wasn't convinced because I'd never seen anyone train like this. Normally, trainers were all about pushing and pain. *I know what I'm doing,* I thought. But he was so sweet that I wanted to go along with what he said just to make him happy. I started listening. I was about to do another rep with the weights when he stopped me. "That's enough, Terry," he said.

"What do we do now?" I asked, looking around the gym.

"That's enough," he said. "Go home. Relax. Let yourself grow."

Of course, relaxing was harder for me than doing almost anything else, especially when I was so anxious about everything in my life. Some nights, Mike invited me over to his house for a simple dinner. It felt good to be out of the hotel, and the conversations we had, along with those workouts, totally changed my mentality. He taught me a new approach that was more about being patient and being kind. And I found that his gentle example inspired me to work harder, so the next day I wanted to lift a little more than I had the day before. He took me to another level, where I was inspired instead of being kicked.

Mike was very cool, peaceful even, but he made me stronger than I'd ever been before. Most of what I learned through him were actually very basic moves—power cleans, dead lifts—but they made me strong. I realized that so much of the other stuff I'd been taught was just fluff, basically people trying to pose and look good for one another. Whereas Mike gave me a basic, positive approach that made me better in everything, and it's been the basis of what I do in the gym ever since.

Finally, I made it to the end of the shoot, and I returned to LA. I was so nervous about seeing Rebecca. I knew I could never tell her my secret. At first, it ate away at my conscience. But then time went by, and I tried to put it out of my mind, until I didn't think about it anymore.

I hadn't gotten fired from my first movie role, and now I was an actor. I actually started getting fairly regular work in movies, and commercials for big brands like Nike and Jack in the Box. But I never gained confidence. And so I used to just kill myself on every role. Even when I had the chance to work with Reginald Hudlin, who'd become like a mentor to me after seeing my film, *Young Boys, Inc.,* I couldn't relax. He put me in a movie called *Serving Sara,* starring Matthew Perry. Because this was my first job acting for Reginald, and he was my friend and my mentor, I pulled him aside, literally, after every scene.

"How was that?"

"How was that?"

"How was that?"

Finally, he wasn't playing anymore.

"Terry, if I said 'cut,' it was good," he said, sounding irritated.

I suddenly got how much I'd been bugging him. I hadn't meant to, but I didn't believe he was telling me the truth when he said I was good. Part of being such an extreme perfectionist was that I never trusted any compliment I was given, and I was always fishing for more. If two people said I did a good job, then I needed five people to say I was good. It could go on to infinity. And, ultimately, it was a losing game. I doubted everything I did. I wanted to be good so badly that I went over my lines until I was delirious. On top of that, I was such a pleaser that I would never make any suggestions to a director or question anything I was told. Even if I wasn't qualified to do a stunt, I did it. I felt like my job was to do whatever I was told, no matter how crazy. "Whatever you tell me, I'll do," I said.

I had spent two years on the TV show *Battle Dome,* and I'd gotten a few movies and commercials in its aftermath. We'd just had our third child. Things were looking really good for us as a family. After having put up with so much over the past ten years, Rebecca was ready to make her first big demand: She wanted a house of our own, which we owned. I did not like this idea from the beginning. I was still bad with money, and I felt like it was enough that we were finally in a rental house we could afford. And I loved that little barn house. It just felt so good to me. But it was clear that, with three kids, we had outgrown our current living space.

"I don't know, Becky," I said. "I just want to sit tight."

"No, Terry, we can buy," she said. "Everybody's buying. We've got to just do it. You're scared."

No man likes to be told he's scared. So that got my attention and dinged my pride. But, even more than that, because of all of the bad decisions I'd made during our marriage, and how much I had put Rebecca through, and my dark secret, I felt like she deserved to finally get something she wanted. I couldn't refuse her.

"You know what?" I said. "Fine."

I still thought it was a bad decision, but I kept my mouth

shut. Rebecca found a pretty house in Pasadena, and our offer was accepted. It was ours. After moving dozens of times in the past twelve years, we had our own home. And then, on the second day after we moved in, all the plumbing went. So I was in this new house, and I couldn't even flush the toilet. The plumber said it was going to cost three thousand dollars for the repair, and I'd spent every penny we had just to buy the house. I had to borrow the money. It was around the holidays, and I couldn't afford anything. We didn't furnish the house. We had nothing.

At least I knew that after the holidays, I'd get back to work on *Battle Dome,* and I'd be able to climb back on top financially. Well, then the show didn't get picked up for another season, and we lost our regular income stream. I wasn't that worried, though. I was getting enough small movie roles and commercials that I knew something would work out. And then there was a commercial strike, and no commercials were being filmed in the city. I didn't have another movie. I didn't have a TV show. I didn't have a commercial, or any hope of landing a commercial anytime soon. And now, for the first time, I had a mortgage. That's when I started to worry.

Our mortgage was only $1,200 a month, but with no income and three kids to support, I couldn't afford even that. All of our creditors started calling the house, and calling the house, and calling the house, and it reminded me of college all over again. I thought I'd seen the end of those dark days, but here I was again. I kept telling myself: *Just concentrate, Terry. Stay focused. Keep doing what you're doing—going to auditions, and writing your own screenplays—and something will come.*

In the middle of all this financial stress, Rebecca got pregnant again, and now we had a new baby on the way. We began to prepare, and I tried to stay positive. And then, in 2002, a few months into Rebecca's pregnancy, she had a miscarriage. It was horrible. We had already been through a miscarriage in college, so I knew how sad it was to lose a baby, but this time it was so much worse. I'm not sure if it was hormones, or stress, or probably a combination of everything, but Rebecca was gone. There were days where she wasn't the same person. She lay in bed, and she couldn't eat. She wouldn't talk to anybody.

When I went into our bedroom and tried to get her to eat a little something, or just make sure she was okay, she talked about strange things that didn't have anything to do with reality, and I worried about her more than ever.

At first, I didn't want to tell anyone what had happened. The miscarriage felt personal, private. I was ashamed of our financial problems, and I didn't want to admit to anyone how bad it had gotten. I felt like all of this was my doing, because of my poor decisions and my dark secret. This was our punishment, and we needed to take it. So I didn't talk to anyone. I just kept my head down and did what needed to be done, which was everything in our house. I made the kids' lunches, took them to school, did the grocery shopping, took care of the house, picked up the kids at the end of the day, got them fed and bathed and into bed.

All the while, I knew we were losing the house. The letters from the bank kept coming and coming. I had no income, and what little money we'd had was gone. I knew there was no way I was going to be able to pay the money we owed on our mortgage. I finally admitted to myself that I had to find us a new place to live.

In ninety days, our house would be gone. My wife was not all there. And I didn't know what to do, so I just prayed: *What should I do?*

And, miraculously, as I prayed, I felt strong. I remembered how, when I was weak and collapsed in on myself, when I thought I hadn't been drafted, when I thought my NFL career was over after the Packers, Rebecca was the one who was strong, and who picked me up and convinced me I had to keep going, no matter what. And now, when she couldn't help herself, I knew I had to be strong for both of us, and I was. Instead of spiraling down into a depression myself, I was able to do what needed to be done at home, and for the kids, and even get myself to auditions. No matter what, I knew I couldn't leave her. And I knew, all over again, that I could never tell her what had happened in Vancouver. I had to keep everything afloat, and I would. But even with all of that, nothing was going to save our house.

CHAPTER 14

BREAK OUT

I WASN'T ABOUT TO ADMIT TO ANYONE, NOT EVEN MY closest friends, how bad things were, and so I hadn't talked to anyone in several months. And then, one day, my phone rang. It was my friend Mark Allenbach. "Hey, Terry, how're you doing?"

"We're doing okay," I said, too proud to admit otherwise.

"Are you up on the house?" he asked.

The question came out of nowhere. I had no idea why he was asking, or how honest I should be. And then, I realized, there was no denying the truth anymore.

"I've got to be out of the house in thirty days," I said. "I'm going to let them take it, man, because right now I can't handle it. I'm looking for a new place to live."

"Look, I'm going to pay what you owe," he said. "We'll put the house up for sale, correctly, and we'll go from there, so you guys can get out in the right way."

"Oh, man," I said.

I didn't know what more to say. I hadn't volunteered any of this information to him. I hadn't asked for help. And yet here he was, offering to save the day.

"I had a feeling that you needed me," he said.

"Thank you."

That was all I could say: Thank you. I was so humbled by his generosity. And I was so grateful that we were going to get a chance to make things right.

Slowly, but noticeably, our circumstances began to turn around. Mark took care of the payments we owed. We put the house up for sale in 2003, and we sold it. We even made a small profit. Mark and I made an agreement that I would pay him $1,000 a month until we were even. This was yet another example of his amazing generosity, because it gave me the chance I needed to get us back on our feet.

At the same time, I knew I had to do something to help Rebecca. I was really worried about her. So I finally called our old pastor Joel Brooks, who had married us back in Kalamazoo. I told him about the miscarriage and the state she'd been in since then.

"I don't know what to do, man," I said. "I mean, what's going on?"

"First of all, take her to a doctor and make sure she's in good health. You've got to get her checked out."

I took Rebecca to be examined, and they realized she had a hormone imbalance following the miscarriage, which had just taken her out. They gave her medicine to regulate her hormones. It also helped that we no longer had the stress of losing the house to worry about. Rebecca started to recover. She got her bearings back, her mood improved, and she came alive. It was such a relief.

I started getting a few small jobs. Rebecca got pregnant

again. Now we really needed a new place to live, but we couldn't afford anything. And then we went to look at a place in Altadena that was so beautiful and well done. After everything we'd been through, I wanted to rent that house for my family, but I knew I didn't have enough money. The owner, Samuel, was from Ghana, and he walked behind Rebecca and me as we looked everything over and then looked at each other.

"So do you want it?"

"Yes, sir."

"I like you. It's yours."

"Well, sir, we've had some issues. I've got some credit stuff."

"I don't need to see credit. I don't need to see anything. I like your spirit. I see you with your wife. I like who you are. You just give me what you can."

It seemed unbelievable, but it was really happening. Rebecca had kept telling me to go for the best place we could. But I'd been feeling bad about myself and all of the mistakes I'd made, so I didn't feel I deserved a nice place. Then I realized this is how faith works: You take action based on where you want to be, not based on where you are. And I began to see that we all get some things in life we don't deserve, and we can all point to times in our lives when things went our way.

Everything was finally good again. But we were still just getting by, and I was hungry to do something to take us to the next level. I had finally landed a part in a movie called *Friday After Next*. I was acting with Katt Williams in most of my scenes, and we became really good friends. He was homeless at the time, and so at the end of the day's shooting, he only pretended to go home. Then he waited until everyone had left and snuck back into his trailer, so no one would know he was living there, and stayed overnight. A few people found out, of course, but they let him do it.

At the same time, I'd been going through everything at home, selling the house, trying to look for a place to live, and not knowing what we were going to do. So Katt and I really bonded, and we made a vow: This could be the last project for both of us, and so we've got to make it memorable. We've got to go all out.

What we did on that movie became the catalyst for so many things that happened for me later in my career. My character was a really despicable guy, and I had nothing to lose, so I threw all of my stress at home into my performance. When we were filming, I was able to completely enter this other character and forget all of my own problems, and that felt so amazing that I just went for it.

The film was a comedy, but I played this big guy who'd just come out of jail and taken a liking to this pimp, played by Katt. We had a scene in a bathroom, where I was pretty much trying to take advantage of him. Well, even though it was a comedy, we played this scene as if it was *The Deer Hunter*. Seriously, if you turned the sound off, so there were no cues to tell you to laugh, it would be horrifying. We were sweating and crying, and he was slapping me, and I think it really added a layer to that film that made it deeper than just a straightforward comedy.

When I took Rebecca to the premiere, she couldn't handle that movie at all, especially when it came time for the bathroom scene.

"Oh, this movie is crazy," she said. "This is not my thing."

"I know, honey," I said. "I know."

But then, there were so many moments when I was on-screen and the theater just erupted. So maybe comedy was for me. When I'd filmed the movie, I'd been in a place where I was so desperate, and as actors, we often find comedy in sadness. So much comedy happens in this strange dark place. It's where Richard Pryor and so many of the comedy greats came from, and I felt all of that when I watched the movie. During one of the worst times in my life, I was able to laugh, and I was able to make other people laugh. And that was a really powerful moment for me.

"Terry, these people are cracking up," Rebecca said during the premiere.

"I know," I said.

This is powerful. This is a very powerful place.

And then, at the after-party, Rebecca rushed up to me, so excited.

"Ice Cube came up to me," she said. "He was like, man, the first two acts, it's me and Mike Epps, and the whole third act is Terry and Katt. They stole the movie."

Ice Cube wasn't the only one who had good things to say. People kept approaching me at the premiere. They were excited. I could feel it coming off them.

N OW THAT THINGS WERE GETTING BACK ON TRACK, Rebecca and I could concentrate on the excitement and joy of the new baby she was carrying. I thought back to my dream about watching my son play football, and I was sure this baby was the boy I had envisioned. But, again, Rebecca told me this baby was a girl, too. Having just come out of the horror of the miscarriage and the loss of our house, and with four girls already at home, I was sure this was it for me, and our family was now complete. I wanted to concentrate on getting back in sound financial shape with the family we already had. My dream had been so vivid that a part of me was disappointed that I would never have a son. But Rebecca assured me that God had promised to send her someone special, and she was absolutely right.

Our little baby Wynfrey was born in 2003, and after such sadness just one year before, she was an absolute treasure. I turned my attention to the newest addition to our family and began to make peace with the fact that the boy I had dreamed about was probably my grandchild. I figured we would be much older when Rebecca held our grandson on the staircase she had envisioned, but I knew we'd be just as happy with the boy in our family's next generation.

I did some other smaller parts in 2003, including a role in Jamie Kennedy's film *Malibu's Most Wanted,* where I played a gang member alongside Damien Dante Wayans. Because of my performance, Damien recommended me to his nephews for a new project they were writing called *White Chicks,* for which they needed an athletic kind of guy. At the same time, Damon Wayans also had a show, *My Wife and Kids,* which was looking for a new regular.

So it worked out that in the morning, I had an audition for *My Wife and Kids,* and in the afternoon, I had an audition for *White Chicks.* Well, let me tell you, I have never bombed during an audition like I bombed that morning. My hands were shaking while I held the paper with my lines on it. Damon and the other producers were looking at one another like they couldn't believe I'd been recommended so highly for the job. Afterward, I got in my car, and I called my agent, even though I almost didn't want to know what they'd said to him.

"How did I do?" I asked.

"Well, we're not hearing anything yet, but go on over to the other audition with Keenen," he said.

I did not want to go. All I could think was how, sometimes, when things start off bad, they tend to go worse. But as I drove across town to the west side of LA, I tried to psych myself up:

Man, I've got nothing to lose. I already stunk up the first deal so bad.
I might as well just go for it.

It was like the exact opposite of what had happened in the morning. I was reading the lines without even looking at the pages. I was doing the part like I *was* that guy, and it was just coming out of me. Keenen Ivory Wayans was cracking up. It was the best audition I've ever done, even to this day. I had that same feeling I'd had trying out for *Battle Dome.* I waited a day and a half, and then my agent called me.

"Good news and bad news," he said. "Bad news, they're going in another direction on *My Wife and Kids.*"

"I knew it because I stunk it up so bad," I said.

"But the good news is you got *White Chicks.*"

Rebecca and I just screamed.

T HAT WAS ONE OF THE BEST PERIODS IN MY LIFE. I WAS actually making money. We were still renting, but the house was great, and we could afford it. I was paying my friend back. The kids were getting older and more acclimated to where they were. Rebecca had totally rebounded, and it felt like we were finally on our way.

But now that I wasn't just in survival mode, I had the chance to take inventory of the many mistakes I'd made along the way, and how close I'd come to ruining everything, especially with what I'd done in Vancouver. Not only were we still standing, but also, we were actually thriving. I was full of hope for what was to come. I vowed never to mess up again, and never to let Rebecca know what I'd done. Now that I understood how close I'd come to losing everything, I was going to hold on tighter than ever.

All of this was very much on my mind because we filmed *White Chicks* in Vancouver, and so I was on location where the stress of my first acting experience had made me go off the rails. I never did so again, but my secret was very present for me while we were there. I thought about how I should really tell Rebecca, but I just couldn't. Things were going too well after they had been so bad for so long. Luckily, my experience on *White Chicks* was so positive that it reversed my first Vancouver nightmare. In fact, filming *White Chicks* was the best experience of my professional life, ever. All of the Wayanses—Keenen, Marlon, Shawn—and producer Rick Alvarez and all of those other guys were so great. And I've never been in the zone quite like that, before or after. I was firing on all cylinders.

I shot my scenes for the film maybe three times a week, and so I had a day or two off between my days on the set. I wanted to be excellent, so I practiced, practiced, practiced. One morning I was working on my dance moves in my room, and the maid walked in on me. I froze, mid-glide.

"Oh, I'm sorry," I said.

Her face said: *Okay, what's going on here?* She laughed and closed the door.

When I had ideas for jokes, I brought them to Keenen.

"Go for it," he said. "Do it."

And so I went for it, again and again, and it all worked. We did the scene where I was singing in the car in one take. And then, it seemed like everything I did was one take. I didn't even have to look at the lines.

"Do you have any notes for me?" I asked.

"Brother," Keenen said. "Just do what you do. No notes. Let's go. Don't stop."

I was almost on a constant high. Here I was, working with my hero, one of the most accomplished comic actors, writers, producers, and directors of all time, the guy who gave us *In Living Color,* Jamie Foxx, J.Lo, and Jim Carrey, and he loved everything I did. "You're killing it," he said. "Man, just go. Just keep going."

When he did give me notes, he shared tips with me about how to do comedy and what it's all about, and where the jokes really hit. I just soaked it all up. And then, Shawn and Marlon were always around, telling me what we were going to do, and it was so smooth, it felt like a family. I felt like a member of the Wayanses.

Everybody kept telling me the same thing: "Terry, this is something special."

After three months of filming in Vancouver, we wrapped. I felt tremendous sadness. I was beginning to understand the problem with being a performer, always chasing the high of performing, and then struggling with the extreme depression that hits after projects are done. When I got home, it was back to reality in a big way.

"The trash is loaded up over there," Rebecca said, pointing.

I looked at her and sighed. I'd just come from nailing every take and being extolled for my talents, to taking out the trash, and it was humbling. It hurt. Honestly, I was mean to my family because I felt like my life had been better in Vancouver when I was filming than it was at home with them. Obviously, looking back, I can see that my perspective was clouded by my depression. But at the time, I was just in it, and I was a jerk.

"You're nicer when you've got a job," my family said.

"I know," I said. "I know."

Rebecca was not about to let me get full of myself, and so she loved to tease me about how it was when I was on location, versus how it was at home.

"I know when you're on the set, it's all, 'Here's your chicken breast, Mr. Crews,' " she said. " 'Here's your smoothie, Mr. Crews.' But, here, it ain't gonna be like that."

But do you have to say it? I know it's not like that at home, but don't say it.

I couldn't wait for the movie to come out. I knew everything was going to be different for me once people got a chance to see it. In the meantime, I lay in bed for hours, and I couldn't make myself get up and do anything.

"Babe, I've got to get back to doing something," I said. "I can't not work."

It was almost like I was addicted to the high of landing my next project and then going on set and achieving that feeling of just nailing it. I was always wondering: *Where's my next job? What's it going to be?*

It was impossible for me to just sit still and feel whatever it was I was going through. As a football player, and the alpha male, I'd adopted this mind-set that was all about blinking through anything bad that happened, and avoiding all negativity at any cost. This rule applied to me, and also to my family: *Don't do anything that will take me down. If you're feeling bad, do something to make yourself feel good.*

Now I know that's the wrong way to be, but at the time, I was acting almost like this horrible, domineering trainer to my wife and kids. And after a while, they didn't want to hear it anymore. Even if they knew I was right, they wouldn't do what I said because of my delivery. My attitude created tension, especially with Azi, who was a teenager. Even when Azi was a youngster, we'd butted heads. One time when she was eight, she did something wrong, and I let her know she was about to get spanked as punishment. She looked at me with this complete and utter calm.

"Dad, you don't ever have to spank me," she said. "Just tell me what to do, and I'll do it."

I was really struck by that moment, but at the time, I was too wrapped up in my own vision of how things needed to be to alter my attitude or approach in any way. Azi was very sensitive, and she was often troubled by the ways of the world. I wasn't sympathetic at all. I didn't want her bringing me down.

"If you're feeling bad, just go play with your toys," I said.

Looking back now, I can see that she was really just looking for somebody to listen to her. Sometimes we have to make the time to sit with the people who are important to us in our lives and feel their pain, open ourselves up enough to acknowledge what feels bad in their lives. Often, that's all people need, is to have their feelings validated, and they'll feel better. But I was a long way from being able to do that at the time. I would not validate anyone's feelings or emotions, especially not my first two kids', because I was the most stunted back then.

I was the super-driven, superstar, alpha male. You can't be manlier than I was. It's just true. I was in the NFL. For my first job in Hollywood, they put me in a cage, and I had to fight other men. I was that guy. And as far as I was concerned, the only emotions people should feel were positive. Anything negative, get it out of here.

Next up, I auditioned for the part of the President Dwayne Elizondo Mountain Dew Herbert Camacho in Mike Judge's *Idiocracy*. I knew this was the follow-up to *White Chicks* that would make me a household name, and I really wanted that part. But it was callback after callback, and my agent wouldn't even tell me who I was up against because he was afraid if I knew my competition, I'd get too psyched out. When I finally got the part, I was overjoyed. Except for one little thing. We were filming in Austin, Texas, during the time when the *White Chicks* premiere happened, and so I wasn't able to attend. Rebecca and the kids went, and I couldn't wait until they got home to give me a report. I called Rebecca while I knew she was still there.

"Terry, the theater is erupting," she said. "I can't believe it. Everybody's coming up to me, like: 'Yo, your husband. Your husband.' Everybody is freaking out. The moment when the scene in the car happened, Terry, they wouldn't stop laughing. The room burst into pandemonium. It was awesome."

"Oh, I wish I was there," I said.

And then the producer, Rick Alvarez, called me, also from the premiere.

"Your life will never be the same," he said. "Everybody is on the floor at everything you're doing. People are going crazy. Get ready, man. This is huge."

Even though I was far away, sitting in my hotel room in Austin, I was so high with endorphins from all of that praise. Also while there, I got a call I'd been waiting on for years. When I'd first moved to Los Angeles, I'd combed the Wilshire Corridor with my head shot and résumé, from one big talent agency to another, only to be told I needed a referral in order to have a meeting. I'd made a promise to myself that I'd be back at one of the premier agencies someday. Meanwhile, around the time I'd done *Malibu's Most Wanted,* a top talent manager, Brad Slater, contacted me to tell me that he saw something special in my performances. He also told me that he couldn't sign me because I was not quite there yet, and I needed to do more first. Honestly, I agreed, but I told him when the time was right, I wanted to be his client. Our positive interaction had always reminded me of Coach Lee's good word that I'd taken all the way to the NFL. Here was a top talent manager telling me he was impressed by my work, and it was a word I'd held on to for years. Now he'd just landed as an agent at William Morris, and he'd immediately gotten me on the phone.

"Hey, TC!" he exclaimed. "It's Brad. Remember when I told you we had to wait until you were ready? I think you're ready!"

And so began a relationship that has only grown stronger over the last ten years. Agents get a bad rap in Hollywood because most artists feel it's an agent's job to get them work, and they're disappointed when that doesn't happen. I've never felt that way. I've always believed it's our job to get the work, and then our agents take everything we're already doing and launch it into the stratosphere. It constantly amazes me how one job I'm already doing so often turns into several new opportunities that presented themselves because my agent knows what he's doing. Brad has always leveraged everything I do into something much bigger and greater, and I believe that's the only way it should be. On top of amazing success, we've seen some crushing disappointments, of course, but stuck with each other the whole way.

Acting is really a confidence game. The more confident you become, the better you are, and I became more and more sure of myself after *White Chicks*. It hit theaters in June 2004 and started doing really well. Not only that, but also, people were talking about my performance. I started getting recognized more and more. I finished *Idiocracy* that summer, and I was waiting for the buzz from *White Chicks* to hopefully bring me something big. I wanted no replay of my experience the year before in *Starsky & Hutch,* where I'd basically been a glorified background player with a name. After the rush of two parts in two major films, I wanted the big time.

But as of Halloween, I was still in between jobs and more than a little unsure about what would happen next. That night was the Harvest Festival at Faith Community Church in West Covina, which Rebecca and I thought would be fun for the kids and a safe way for the little ones to get candy without going door to door. And it was. As we loaded everyone into the car at night's end, Rebecca turned to me.

"Can you help me get Wynfrey from her stroller into her seat?"

This was an odd request since Wynfrey was less than a year old at the time and certainly not too big for Rebecca to carry, but I didn't say anything about it. I snapped Wynfrey into her car seat, helped the other kids climb in, and then hopped into the driver's seat. As I did, I said what came into my mind, almost as a joke.

"Why can't you put the kids in? What are you, pregnant?"

Deafening silence.

My head whipped around to look at Rebecca as a sweet smirk snuck onto her face. Whoa, I hadn't been serious, but THIS was serious.

"Becky, are you pregnant?"

Staring out the front window, she nodded: YES.

My mouth dropped open. My head filled with a million thoughts at once.

"Really?"

As if the answer would change if I asked again. She looked at me and smiled.

"Yes, I'm pregnant."

My mood was bittersweet. I was ecstatic that we were bringing another life into the world, but I was filled with dread at the prospect of trying to afford five kids in LA with the insecurity of an actor's transient life and uncertain income. I knew we had faithfully used contraception every time. Even as I saw disappointment cross Rebecca's face, I couldn't hide my fear. I took a deep breath.

"Are you sure?"

"I took a pregnancy test twice because of how I've been feeling lately," she said. "And they both came up positive."

Finally, I had worked my way through my shock and anxiety, and I was able to just be happy. I smiled at her and hugged her right there in the front seat. We grinned at each other: *Here we go again!*

A few months later, I accompanied Rebecca to her ultrasound. After our second miscarriage, I was feeling extremely anxious. I wanted everything to go smoothly, and I felt my presence at the appointment would be good for both of us. The nurse rubbed the gel on Rebecca's belly and began moving the instrument across her skin. It didn't take long for her to turn to us and smile.

"Do you want to know the sex of the baby?"

I looked at Rebecca. Now, I was fairly certain we were going to have another girl, because it was said that fathers tend to have a run on the same sex in families of more than three children. Rebecca, however, had told me from the beginning that this baby was a boy. She could feel it. Rebecca and I smiled at each other.

"Yes," we both said.

"You've got a boy," the nurse said.

She showed us a little mark on the ultrasound that let her know for sure, and with that, I knew my dream and Rebecca's vision were no coincidence.

WAS GETTING SMALL JOBS HERE AND THERE, BUT NOTHING steady. Rebecca was always telling me that even though I thought I was a movie guy, I needed to do some TV, especially now that we had our fifth kid on the way.

"Yeah, I don't know if I'm a TV guy," I said. "I don't know if everybody wants to see me every day."

"Yeah, but you need to try it," she said. "You need to see."

Now, by this point, I was starting to see that Rebecca had always been the voice of wisdom in our relationship, especially when it came to my career. She'd gotten me out to Los Angeles in the first place. So when I got the call to go in and do a guest spot on *My Wife and Kids,* I was more than ready to give it a try. I was also happy to be back with the Wayans family again. I still thought of *White Chicks* as one of the best acting experiences of my life, and I wanted to redeem myself after I'd botched my first audition for the show. Plus, I'd never really done true episodic television, and I was eager to see what it was all about.

Let me tell you, it was nothing like what I'd expected. In the first three days, I did a table read, a minor walk-through, and a camera walk-through, and Damon wasn't on set for any of this. I couldn't figure out how it was going to work when the cameras started rolling. I'd really liked the script as it was written, but I had an idea for how I thought it could be even better, and after how well my ad-libbing had gone during *White Chicks,* and also *Idiocracy,* I felt empowered to speak up. Damien was sitting with some of the other writers, and I approached them.

"Have you ever had a trainer who was not interested in getting you in shape at all?" I asked. "He just wanted to show you that you could never do what he does?"

"Oh, yeah," Damien said, already laughing.

"I see this guy like that," I said. "What would happen if I take Damon through these things, and he can't do any of them?"

The way it was written, he did everything, and then he got really sore.

"In fact, better than that, not only can't he do any of it, but I can do it ten times better than he does."

When we did the final camera walk-through, I showed them some of the things I was thinking about. They were laughing so hard, they decided to change the whole script. I went home that night, and when I came back on Thursday, which was the tape day, I still didn't know if we were going to do it as it had originally been written, or if we were going to try it my way. Well, they had totally rewritten the script, and it was so cool because that really improved my confidence.

I can do this, I thought. Up until then, I'd always felt a bit like I was still a football player, and I didn't really know what this acting world was all about, and so I should just keep my mouth shut and do what I was told. But here I was in a whole new style of comedy, doing this multi-camera sitcom, which I had never done before. And, maybe, I was good at it.

When the camera started rolling, Damon and I just went for it, and it was pure magic. We were in the zone. My name was Darryl, a gym employee who specialized in EuroTraining, which was this psychotic style of working out. Damon was making things up off the top of his head, and I was bouncing off of him, and finally, it was a whole new episode. When it was done, it was just like *White Chicks* had been, but in a TV show format. That experience changed something for me. *I can do this,* I thought. The world seemed to agree. That episode aired in late 2004, and it has always been considered one of the best episodes of *My Wife and Kids*. It currently has more than six million hits on YouTube, which made that one TV show as big as anything else I'd ever done at that point.

CHAPTER 15

THAT'S NOT HOW IT'S DONE

AT THIS POINT, I WAS REALLY RECEPTIVE TO television, especially with another baby on the way. I'd also started to get frustrated with how a movie experience would be really great, but then I'd have to wait a year for the film to come out. And then, sometimes, it would get buried, like had happened with *Idiocracy,* which had opened in only seven theaters in its first weekend. I'm still not exactly sure what happened with that film. But I was told there was a huge blowback against the studio because we had jokes on everyone from Costco to Carl's Jr., who had all thought they were getting product placements, until they realized they were getting punked instead. At the time, I was devastated that so few people got to see that film.

I was approached about doing a new TV show, and I was open to it, so we entered into discussions. It felt like maybe I was starting to get a little light as a performer. Around the same time, I auditioned for the Adam Sandler comedy *The Longest Yard*. Since it was a football movie, and I was one of the few former NFL players working in Hollywood, I thought maybe there was something in the film for me. They kept trying me out for all of these different roles, but they didn't know what they wanted. And then, one day, I got a call from my agent, Brad.

"Dude, you're about to get a call from Adam Sandler right now," he said. "Keep your phone on. He wants to talk to you. It's about *The Longest Yard*. I know we had you bouncing around to different roles, but he's got it now."

Let's just say it's hard to do anything else when you're waiting for a career-making call from Adam Sandler. I sat and stared at my phone. Finally, there he was.

"Hey, buddy, how you doing?" he said.

"Hey," I said, while thinking: *THIS IS ADAM SANDLER*.

"Hey, man, check it out, you killed me in *White Chicks*. It's the funniest thing I've ever seen. I've got this role for you. We want you to play Cheeseburger Eddy."

Now, in the script, Cheeseburger Eddy was a 300-pound guy, like Fat Albert.

"But I'm not obese," I said.

"Nah, nah, nah, what we're going to do is you're muscular, you're in shape, and you're eating cheeseburgers," he said. "That's even better."

"All right," I said.

"Dude, you're in, you're Cheeseburger Eddy," he said. "I love it, man. I'll see you on the set. You're in."

I went to Santa Fe, New Mexico, to shoot *The Longest Yard,* and this was another dream project for me. First of all, it was a superstar cast. Chris Rock was costarring, and it had everyone in it. Even better, I felt like this was my revenge on the NFL. I was going to show them that I hadn't just disappeared. I was back, and career-wise, I was better than ever. The film also re-united me with my old teammate from the Rams, Bill Gold-berg, who'd become a wrestling superstar after his time in the NFL. That was so great, and Bill is one of the best people you could ever know.

Even then, with things going so well, I could not break my addiction to porn. When I went away on location, I watched adult movies on pay-per-view in my hotel room, even as I vowed to stop. But when Friday night rolled around, I couldn't resist the temptation. Then I threw myself into my performances and workouts even more in order to make up for my guilt. Let me tell you, it was an exhausting way to live.

Filming *The Longest Yard* was another incredible experi-ence, on par with *White Chicks*. It felt like being away at sum-mer camp. I was working with my heroes, and everyone was having the best time. I was getting paid. The food was good and abundant. I'd been starving on and off for the past six years, and here I was, in heaven once again. And best of all, everything I did for the camera was working: riffing off the other actors, doing crazy stuff, dancing. Adam was laughing so hard. "Put that in the movie," he said. "That's in the movie."

Chris Rock and I developed a friendship, and he was coming up with stuff off of what I was doing. He looked at me dancing one day and it just came out: "That's a big-ass robot," he said.

Everyone was just dying, they were laughing so hard.

While I was on the set, it was Tera's birthday, and so Becky brought all of the kids to visit so we could celebrate together. I pulled Rebecca aside.

"Look at our lives, Becky," I said. "Look, can you believe it?"

She shook her head, smiling so big. That whole visit, she and I were always looking at each other, giving each other double takes, like: *Look what we're doing.*

I could see Chris noticing that I was a family guy, and while we were on the set together he started asking me questions about being a husband and a dad, but I didn't think much of it. After the film was finished, we were all invited to the Super Bowl as part of the film's promotion. With Adam Sandler's production company, the Happy Madison clan, the way they do everything is just enormous—limo buses, and tickets for everybody, and all of these amazing events. The whole time, Chris was watching me and asking questions.

"So, yeah, how long you been married?"

"Sixteen years in July."

"How many kids you got?"

"Four."

He just kept going, but again, I wasn't really thinking about his questions because it was so amazing to finally be at the Super Bowl. After all my years of struggle in the NFL, and then in Hollywood, now, finally, I felt like I'd found where I belonged. As we were leaving the Super Bowl, Chris pulled me aside one last time.

"Terry, I've got something for you," he said. "I can't tell you about it now," he said. "I can't tell you, but I've got it. I've got it. Just wait for it."

Wow, I thought. *Chris Rock says he's got something for ME.*

I loved making movies. I wanted to make more movies. When it went well, it was this absolute high. It was what I wanted to do for the rest of my life. After the fun I'd had working with the Wayanses on *My Wife and Kids,* I was open to TV. But when I thought about doing it instead of movies, a part of me was like: *Do I have to?*

As usual, Rebecca was the smart one in our family.

"Honey, you've got to do TV because TV is going to be the thing for you," she said. "And it gives us security."

Yeahhh, security-smurity, I thought. (Remember, this was the before part.)

"I'm loving being away on film sets, though," I said.

"But we need you to be able to come home at night," she said. "And if you do a good show, it will provide everything we need."

Inside, I was still the risk taker, but after sixteen years of her good advice mostly keeping us from being taken down by the disasters I'd set in motion, I got it.

"I'm listening," I said. "You're right. I've got to get a TV show. I've got to do something like that."

In the midst of all this, there was that television show I'd been offered. I was still not quite ready to commit, but I'd been told I had to give them a decision by the end of the day, and everything was telling me that I needed to move toward TV.

That day, a messenger delivered a script to the house. I opened it up, expecting it to be a revised script for the show I was in discussions about, but the title read *Everybody Hates Chris.* No one had told me it was coming, so I had no idea what to expect. It was the funniest thing I'd read in years. It was genius, so well done it was like a half-hour movie all about Chris's life as a little boy. They wanted me to play his dad. On top of that, my old mentor and friend Reggie Hudlin was directing the pilot, and he'd also recommended me for the part.

Now, he and I hadn't really been in touch since he'd backed out of producing my film, *Young Boys, Inc.,* after he'd directed me in *Serving Sara.* Before I moved to Los Angeles, I'd cut a trailer of my film so I could shop it around to potential investors for completion funds. I gave it to everyone who would take it and met with rappers, actors, music producers—anyone I thought might be interested. Once I got to LA, a friend took the trailer videocassette to his barbershop and asked the guys there what they thought. The reaction was pretty good overall, but more important, Reginald Hudlin was in the barbershop at the time, saw the trailer, and loved it. Reginald had directed *House Party,* and *Boomerang* with Eddie Murphy, and eventually went on to produce *Django Unchained* with Quentin Tarantino. The funny thing was, I'd just been in his office the day before he saw my trailer, hoping to get a copy of it to him. But his assistant, Traci Blackwell, who was very good at her job, blocked me hard. My initial rejection made it all the sweeter when Reggie gave his card to my friend to set up a meeting. I then went back to his office and smiled at Traci as I told her Reggie wanted to meet with me now. She gave me a little side-eye, conferred with Reggie, and let me into his office. Traci is now a vice-president of current programming at the CW Network. I told you she did her job well.

Reggie was the first person to show me what real Hollywood was about. Even while I was doing security, he invited my family and me to parties at his gorgeous home in Beverly Hills. He was one of the smartest men in the business, and I met so many great people through him. In fact, the first time I ever met Arnold Schwarzenegger was when Reggie invited me to dinner with him. Reggie also invited me to movie premieres such as *Mission: Impossible 2,* where I rubbed shoulders with John Woo and Tom Cruise. Sometimes Reggie screened movies at his home theater, and I sat dumbfounded at how cool it was when he pressed a button and the screen descended from the ceiling. His home looked like a museum, with marble everywhere inside, and bougainvillea all over the exterior. Vintage movie posters from thirties- and forties-era black cinema covered the walls. All of this, and yet he continued to hang with a struggling security guard with dreams of making it in Hollywood. I always told myself: *Once I make it, that's how I want to be.*

So it had been very painful for me when my talks with Reg-

gie about working together on *Young Boys, Inc.,* didn't come to
fruition. My agent at the time hadn't handled the situation well,
and I'd been so hungry to get something going that my feelings
had been hurt. I wasn't mad at Reginald, but it stung. And then
I got busy just trying to keep afloat, and he and I hadn't spoken
in several years. So it felt amazing to be back in the fold with
him. As soon as we reconnected, it was like old times again. I
will always have so much respect for him.

Reginald shot the pilot for *Everybody Hates Chris,* and then
there was this nervous energy around everything while we
waited to see if we were going to get picked up. I wanted it so
badly. We got word that we were being flown to New York for
the upfronts, which was when the new shows are pitched to ad-
vertisers, and was a good sign that we'd gotten picked up.

Finally, it was official: We had been picked up. And that was
yet another best day of my life so far. Not only was the show a
go, but also, this little UPN sitcom was the most highly touted
pilot of the year. It felt so great.

That morning, Chris and I stood onstage together at Madison Square Garden, waving at everybody and just beaming with
joy. That night was the Los Angeles premiere for *The Longest
Yard.* So Chris and I hopped on CBS's private jet and flew from
New York to LA, to attend the premiere with Adam Sandler.
As soon as he saw me at the premiere, he came up and gave me
a big hug.

"Hey, buddy," he said. "We did it, buddy."

My feet did not touch the ground that entire day. Everything
we'd endured to get there played through my mind, and I had
the thought that even during the moments that are the darkest
of the dark, we should never kill ourselves because there's something amazing on the other side. Here I was, living my dream,
and I knew my life would once again never be the same.

The network did a huge takeover to launch *Everybody Hates Chris*. We were on billboards and every bus in New York City. We were on the cover of *Entertainment Weekly*. It was epic. *This is what it feels like,* I thought.

We also worked really, really hard. I decided to get my sports mentality on and never rest on the assumption that we were good. I was determined to be beyond great. I really wanted to show Chris what I could do and thank him for giving me this kind of opportunity. And because the part was based on Chris's father, who had not lived to see his success, I wanted to really honor that memory and role.

Rebecca was right there. "I told you, TV is the way," she said. "I told you."

"I know," I said. "You are always right."

And she hadn't just been right about TV, either. In December 2005, after we shot our first thirteen episodes of *Everybody Hates Chris,* we rented a five-bedroom house in a gated community in Altadena, California. It was the biggest house we'd ever lived in, palatial compared to anywhere else we'd stayed. Just before Christmas, Rebecca stood on the staircase, holding our little six-month-old boy, Isaiah, and we realized that her vision had come true.

Now that we'd made it, I had some ideas about what this meant. I was going to buy Rebecca a new car. So I made her trade in her car, which she loved, and I got her a huge black Escalade. It had rims and tinted windows and everything.

"This is the car you want," I said.

She thanked me, but she never seemed that excited about her new car, and I couldn't understand why. I had picked it for her, done everything, and she just didn't seem to appreciate it. I was hurt, and I sat for hours, pouting about how ungrateful she was. Let me tell you, back then, I could get into a pity party, with the pointy hat and the blower and everything. I mean I've had pity parties that rivaled New Year's Eve, but the thing about the pity party is that no one else ever comes to your pity party. Not that I didn't try. I talked to many of my guy friends and got them to agree.

"Yeah, dude, what's wrong with her?" they said.

I couldn't figure it out.

I always had plenty to say when Rebecca did something I wasn't happy with, though. For example, my wife could not cook a great meal due to how picky I was about whatever she did. Because I was that critical of myself, I picked her apart, instead of just appreciating the fact that she'd made a hot meal for my family and me. Whatever she did, I always gave her a grade, and I felt fine with that. As far as I was concerned, hey, I get graded at work, and so she had to get graded at home. Instead of having the mentality that we were a team that was working together to make a home and raise our family, I acted as if I was her boss.

It was the same way with my oldest daughters, now that they were teenagers. I always wondered why I was having problems with my family during those years. We could finally stop worrying about money and stress and just relax and enjoy everything, but somehow, we fought more than ever.

One day, Naomi finally faced me. "You can't control me, Dad," she said.

"What are you talking about?" I said. "Nobody's trying to control you. I'm providing for you. That's just what this is. You're living in my house."

It led to a big rift. We were always arguing about something, and she'd finally left home when she was just fifteen years old. At that moment, I didn't have the clarity to be the adult in that situation, and I was just done with our relationship.

Of course, I was hardest of all on myself. I was incredibly controlling, and it created a tremendous amount of anxiety within me because I was often trying to rule aspects of life that were beyond my control. I tried to bend the world to my will, tried to make things happen, tried to make people like me. If the weather was gray, I wanted to turn it into sunshine. Now I can see that this went back to the lack of control I experienced when I was a kid. But at the time, I didn't understand anything, and all I knew was how anxious I felt, all of the time, even at moments like this when my life was actually going incredibly well. Even when my agent, and my directors, and my costars reassured me again and again that I was doing a good job, and my career was going well, I couldn't believe them. When people told me they loved my performance, I didn't believe they were telling me the truth. Because I was always trying to control others, I believed they were also trying to control me, and their compliments were attempts to manipulate me.

My paranoia warped everything. Even while I was doing *Everybody Hates Chris,* which was by all accounts a very successful show, I became dissatisfied with my own performances. I didn't feel good about what I was doing or how it was being received. I should have been having the time of my life. I loved working with Chris and Reginald. I'd also been unexpectedly reunited with another old friend when Devon Shepard was hired as a staff writer. It had been years since he wrote for *The Fresh Prince of Bel-Air,* and I was an NFL player, and we marveled at our life paths.

"Can you believe I'm writing for a show you're starring in?" he asked.

"I know!" I said.

At the same time, I had a head-on-collision with the show's cocreator and producer, Ali LeRoi. He believed the world revolved around him. And I believed the same about myself at the time, even though I felt like I was able to keep it off of the set. Let's just say that when these two viewpoints collided, it didn't work. Because it was his world, and he'd created it, everything had to go down the way he chose, and this led to many problems.

I often had my lines memorized and all worked out, and then at the last second, Ali changed everything. I tried to reframe my experience and understand that being forced to think on my toes would make me a better actor, but it was exhausting. And then the creative tensions on the set flared up to the point during the second season where Devon left the show, and that really hurt me.

"Man, I wish I could stick it out here for you, brother," he said. "Can't do it."

I knew it was nothing personal between Devon and me, but that was my heart, and his departure made it impossible for me to respect Ali. At the time, if a person did me wrong, even once, that was it, we were done. Given the childhood I'd had, trust was something I hadn't had the luxury of developing. The same was true of standing up for myself, which I'd always felt there was no point in doing when I knew the other person wasn't going to listen to me anyhow.

Instead, what I had mastered was the art of avoiding and moving on from many people who'd been very close to me, rather than simply telling them that they'd done something I didn't like. I was ready to make that move with Ali, and I was ready to do it with the show. But then something remarkable happened.

Realizing the show's future was in jeopardy, the producers spoke to Ali, and he asked me to sit down with him in the commissary. I did not have high hopes for that conversation. But he spoke simply and from the heart, and he vowed to change. And then he did. That was huge for me. It made me realize that people can change. Maybe he only made the shift for business purposes, but I didn't really care, as long as I felt respected. I'd needed to start giving people a second chance, and Ali was the first time I did so in my life. The fact that the results were so positive made me think that maybe I could do it again. The last two years of *Everybody Hates Chris* went well.

That was an amazing time for me. I was invited over to Eddie Murphy's house by a friend to watch a boxing match. I couldn't believe it. Eddie Murphy was a megastar, one of those guys who changed entertainment forever, and I was going to his house! My friend picked me up, and we drove to a gated neighborhood in Beverly Hills. I was incredibly nervous when the guard looked at me like he wasn't going to let me through. But then, a few seconds later, we were on the other side.

It was like rolling through the gates of heaven. Giant sculptured lampposts adorned the streets. Every home we passed was so grand and tasteful that each could probably fit five or six McMansions inside. We pulled up to his house and encountered another huge gate, where my friend stated his name into the intercom on the driver's side.

The gates opened inward, and I was shocked to see that we were driving over a stone bridge straddling an actual stream that was connected to a waterfall that mysteriously emanated from the house. We parked in the driveway, and I gaped at the Mercedes, Lamborghinis, and Bentleys that sat in full view.

The closer we drew to the house, the more nervous I became. Eddie's assistant greeted us. He was as cool as could be, and he invited us in and asked if we wanted something to drink. I could hardly close my mouth because the house looked like the interior of a grand mall, with a living room roof that could open wide on a sunny day. I followed the guys into the kitchen, where champion boxer Sugar Ray Leonard was sitting and talking to MLB all-star Barry Bonds. Arsenio Hall was there and gave me one of the warmest greetings I've ever received from a celebrity. The house was full of people who were accustomed to being there, and who clearly made themselves at home, but I was too nervous.

Someone grabbed a remote, and a flat-screen television rose out of a cabinet with every movie known to man listed on the display, and this was in the days before Netflix. The chatter was fairly boisterous until, all of a sudden, Eddie himself stood at the top of the staircase that led down to the kitchen. *Oh my God, there he is,* I thought. Silence from everyone. They must have been thinking the same thing.

Eddie wore a white Muhammad Ali Adidas tracksuit and slippers, and he scanned the crowd as he descended the stairs. After shaking hands with several people, he looked over at me with an inquisitive look on his face. All I could think was: *Uh-oh, maybe he doesn't want me here.*

Then he made a beeline for me, and now I was certain my assumption was correct. But when he finally stood in front of me, he cracked a slight smile.

"My brother Charlie and I are writing a movie. We've got a part we are writing with you in mind. You wanna be in this movie with us?"

I smiled from ear to ear.

"I sure would! I'd be honored to work with you, brother!"

"I'll get you the script when it's finished," he said, smiling at me again.

I can't believe my life, I thought.

I hung out there for the rest of the day, and Eddie himself

gave me a tour of his home. There was an actual movie theater with a poster showing the times when several first-run movies would be showing. In his house. Wine cellar, bowling alley, school classrooms for the kids, it was all so incredible. He took us up to the roof, where we could see the Los Angeles skyline. The whole time, I told myself: *Nod and don't say anything, so you don't say anything stupid.* We stood overlooking the homes of Samuel L. Jackson, Rod Stewart, and Magic Johnson. I asked him with a neighborhood full of the world's richest, most distinguished people, if their families ever got together. He laughed.

"We have barbecues and try to act normal, but everybody here can only act normal for so long," he said with more laughter. "Then you're reminded that some of these guys haven't flipped a burger in twenty-five years."

Then he naturally did his guttural Eddie Murphy laugh, the one that's entertained millions. I got goose bumps. It was a day I'll never forget.

The film Eddie and Charlie were writing was *Norbit,* and playing that role was one of the most enjoyable experiences to ever happen to me. I played Big Black Jack, brother to a beast of a woman, Rasputia, played by Eddie. Watching him become another person was a marvel, and I still believe the world has not seen a better actor and comedian. Career-wise, I felt like: Wow, this was *that* major moment for me.

At the same time, Rebecca was struggling with how my newfound celebrity had changed my behavior. I started dressing better. I was into my look, and always in front of the mirror. She came up behind me before we went out.

"Is my skin okay?" I asked.

"What are you talking about?" she said.

And then, I turned it on her, and what she was wearing.

"No, no, no, those glasses are not the right kind of glasses," I said. "You've got to wear this other brand instead."

"Stop already," she said.

One day, before a party, I changed three times and the outfit I ended up in was very form-fitting. She looked at me and shook her head in disbelief.

"So you're trying to be all actorly and Mr. Whatever now?"

"Well, yeah," I said. "You know, yeah, I am."

We went to the party, and I actually walked around wearing my sunglasses inside, with this swagger, smoking one of these cigars they were giving out, thinking to myself: *I'm going to act like a star.* When someone talked to me, I blew my smoke right at them and didn't listen to a word they said, thinking the whole time about what I was going to say and how fabulous and hilarious it was going to be.

Rebecca slid away from me. When I found her, I reached for her hand.

"You know what?" she said, pulling away. "You just go and walk around. I'm going to stay right here. Whatever show you're doing, you do it over there."

And I did, I walked around like an idiot—only, at the time, I thought I was Mr. Cool.

When we were in the car driving home, she broke it down for me.

"Honey, I don't know what that was, but I'm not going out with that again."

"Why? What? I'm Hollywood now. See, I'm doing it."

"No, Boo Boo," she said, which she's always loved to do. "That's not how it's done. You gonna be that, I'm at home. Forget that."

I was so lucky to have her. As soon as I played that night back in my head I knew it was fake. And I was embarrassed.

I'm telling you, I'm embarrassed to this day. So I vowed, never again. From then on, I knew I always needed to just be me.

There was one change that I wasn't about to give up, though, because it was actually about becoming the real me I'd always wanted to be but had never been able to finance before then. I could afford to not wear sweats all of the time, and so I made a huge push to finally revamp my wardrobe. I was introduced to a man named Nana Boateng, and Nana changed my life. He's one of the best menswear designers in the world, and one of my good friends. We sit and talk about clothes and fashion for hours.

At first Rebecca had a problem with my new fashion consciousness, because she looked at it as a threat and a sign that I might be looking to step out on our marriage. Otherwise, she couldn't figure out why I was turning into this fashion plate when she hadn't seen me care about this stuff before.

"My thing was always that the kids had what they need," I said, "and you had what you need, but now that we have a little extra, I'm changing my wardrobe."

Even when I explained myself, she didn't like it. She couldn't shake the feeling that I wanted to attract women or was trying to be this Hollywood guy. Honestly, that was not on my mind at all. For me, when it came to fashion, I'd always experienced the same frustration as when I'd painted a picture that did not match the image in my head. So what I decided during *Everybody Hates Chris* was, now that I had a little more money, I was going to dress how I saw myself in my head.

My grand fashion unveiling happened in 2008 at the premiere for *Get Smart,* which I'd acted in along with Steve Carell, Anne Hathaway, Dwayne Johnson, and Alan Arkin. Going into the opening night, Nana let me know he had something special planned. I was excited but also nervous. The thing about fashion, especially because I was just getting a name for myself, was that I'd seen how mistakes stayed with a star forever. But I knew if I didn't do anything, I was missing a great opportunity.

"Okay, Nana, I'm going to get ignored at the premiere," I said. "We have to do something amazing to make sure I'm seen, and I get my turn on the red carpet."

"I've got just the plan," he said.

He made me a three-piece salmon suit that looked pink. Now, this was avant-garde, as far as the color went, but the cut was very European, very classy. It fit wonderfully, and it was just this beautiful suit. But it was pink. I'm an artist, but even I was like: *Wow, can I do this? I don't want people saying I look like a fool.*

And then I reframed it. I'd always gone against the grain. Did I want to live my whole life just being that normal dude, or did I want to keep living an exceptional life? If I got on this red carpet wearing a typical blue suit, and I got ignored, I'd regret it for the rest of my life. "Nana, let's go," I said.

Even though I'd talked myself up, we were girding our loins. This was either going to work, or it was going to fail so hard. When I stepped out of the car, all of the movie's big stars were already on the red carpet, I mean, Dwayne Johnson, Steve Carell, all of them, the cameras literally pulled off of them and went right for me. FLASHES POPPING. EVERYWHERE. *Entertainment Tonight* stopped me to talk about my suit. I'd done other red carpets before, but I'd never gotten that kind of light.

It worked, and I was hooked. I got it after that. Clothing is powerful. It's not that it makes you, but it changes the way people perceive you. From then on, I decided I had to make sure this was part of the game. And I think every man needs to do so in whatever way works for him. Of course, fashion starts inside, and not just with fitness and your body, but also with self-love, but it's all tied together, and it all helps. When we wear something that looks great on us, or something we feel good in, which is even more important, our whole image of ourselves changes.

CHAPTER 16

D-DAY

OT LONG AFTER *EVERYBODY HATES CHRIS* ENDED, in early 2009, I was driving back from a meeting, when I got a dream phone call. It was Robi Reed, who was not only a very famous casting agent, but she'd also cast many films for my longtime hero, Spike Lee, including my favorite, *Do the Right Thing*. By this point, she was working at BET, and she knew the show hadn't been picked up for another season.

"I just wanted to know if you'd be open to meeting with us at BET about a reality show," she said.

I didn't know what to say. As much as I respected and admired her, it seemed like a reality show meant the death knell for most celebrity marriages. When I talked to Brad, he wasn't much more encouraging.

"You know, you've got to be really careful because you could kill your career if they see you as a reality guy," he said. "They could stop calling."

I knew he was right. The hard truth was that, many times, people on reality shows were done with their careers, and here I was, on the rise. The timing did seem off. On the other hand, reality TV was not going away, and I was reading a lot of books just then on the importance of not just doing the norm, because everything is always changing, and if you keep your frame of mind in the past, you can never grow. If there was one thing I knew I wanted to do, it was grow, constantly, forever.

"You know, Brad, I want to try it," I said. "If we do it right, it could work for me. Now, there are a lot of ways it could go wrong, but there are a lot of ways it could go right, too. Plus, if I do it, they have to pay me. I'm not doing *Everybody Hates Chris* anymore, and I need to work, you know, so what's the problem?"

I did have another show in the works at the time, *Are We There Yet?* If it came through, it would be my first starring role, but the negotiations were proving to be long and drawn out, and it was certainly not a sure thing at the moment.

I was able to make Brad see my point. Now I had to convince Rebecca.

"Becky, what do you think about doing a reality show?"

"No way, Terry," she said. "I'm not getting on that camera."

"Okay, cool, I'll tell them," I said. "But I'm just saying, this could be a big deal. I mean, I don't know, could we just meet with them?"

We met with BET, and they told us, immediately, that they wanted to green-light a show about my family and me. If they'd said no, in a way it would have been easier—problem solved— but now I went back to Rebecca.

"Please," I said. "I think this is a good thing. I think we have to look at these opportunities as God sent them to us. *Everybody Hates Chris* is gone. We don't know if *Are We There Yet?* is going to happen."

"I can't do it," she said. "I can't."

"Listen, Becky, I really feel that if you don't do it, you're going to regret it for the rest of your life. You were the one that was in front of the cameras, long before I was. You're the actress. You're the singer. You're the performer. If you allow people to know who you are, and everyone can see how beautiful you are, and what a great mom you are, you're going to win a lot of people over for whatever else you want to do. If you don't want to do it, I hear you, but I think we should do it."

"Ugh."

Well, she slept on it, and she woke up with a new perspective. "Terry, you're right," she said. "I imagined not doing it, and I think I would regret it."

So we got the house ready, and suddenly, it was the night before they were coming over to start filming. She hadn't slept the night before, and she was a wreck.

"Tell them I can't do it," she said. "I can't do it."

I didn't want to cancel, but I could tell she was really serious, so I picked up the phone to make the call.

"No, no, we should do it," she said.

It was back and forth like that all day until I finally had an idea.

"Let's just do the pilot," I said.

Well, she had a ball. We all did. I had always worked without my family, and now, here I was, filming with my wife and all of my kids every day, and I loved it.

Shooting the pilot for our very own reality show, *The Family Crews,* had gone well, and talks were moving forward on *Are*

We There Yet? But in the meantime, I wasn't working, and I'd had a series of letdowns that had made me feel like I had to start making opportunities for myself. When I'd heard they were shooting a remake of *The A-Team,* I knew the part of B. A. Baracus would be perfect for me. I wanted that part so badly, I paid an effects house to create a new interpretation of the character with these spikes in his head, and I made a video of myself in the role, which I then delivered to the producers. When they passed on me, I was devastated. (Never mind that in the past five years, that video has since garnered 600,000 views on You-Tube; the mysteries of casting are not for me to attempt to unravel.) No other big parts had materialized, so I started writing a character called Squeegee, who'd gone from poor window washer to the world's best dancer. I was doing everything in my power to move that project forward, writing and rewriting the script, doing all of the choreography, and doing live dance performances all over LA. I was even using the character for a series of commercials to promote LA public transportation, and I was in a meeting for this latest job, all Squeegeed out, when Brad called.

"Sylvester Stallone wants to meet with you. Right now."

"What are you talking about?"

"Check it out. You've got to get down there. I showed him your video."

"Squeegee?"

This was real. Why would he want to meet with me about Squeegee?

"No, no, I showed him your video of your *A-Team* audition."

Now, at the time, Sly Stallone was making the first *Expendables* movie. He'd already hired Forest Whitaker, but Forest had to drop out. When he went to several other people, he couldn't get anyone interested because the movie wasn't a big deal at the time. Stallone was in his sixties, and when he told everyone he was going to make an action movie, they all laughed at him, and every studio turned him down. He was forced to go to a B player, Millennium Films, which was known for straight-to-video releases. All he had lined up at that point were Jet Li and Jason Statham. But Sly's a force of nature, so he was making calls and doing everything himself, which was how he saw my video and decided he had to meet me.

"Wherever you are," Brad said. "Get to Beverly Hills right now."

Once in Beverly Hills, I found the address, a small office right off of Little Santa Monica. This redheaded kid brought me upstairs into this dim room. And then I heard the voice: gravelly, unmistakable, the one, the only, Sly Stallone.

"Hey, sit down," he said.

It was really weird, almost spooky, and then the lights suddenly went on, and there he was. He sat down across from me.

"I'm doing this movie," he said. "We're shooting it in Brazil. It's going to be pretty good. I've seen some stuff from you."

What I later found out was that he has daughters, and through them and a friend, he'd seen *White Chicks* and really liked it. But all I knew at the time was that he'd seen my audition for the *A-Team* movie, and now he was explaining the project as if he was pitching the movie to me. Meanwhile, I was thinking this was an audition and wondering where the lines were. I wasn't prepared for him to talk to me as if I already had the part.

So I did what I'd done the first time I went to Eddie Murphy's house: Just nod and don't say anything, so you don't say the wrong thing.

"We're going to go down to Brazil," he said. "We're going to have a good time. We'll take care of you. We feel like it would be a real good thing for you."

I just smiled and nodded and tried not to mess it up.

"Let me show you what you're going to be shooting," he said, showing me videos of this amazing, fully automatic shotgun, the AA-12, known as the world's deadliest. "This is your gun in the movie," he added with a smirk.

This is not an audition, I thought. *He's giving me this part, like right now.*

The whole thing didn't take longer than twenty or twenty-five minutes, and let me tell you, I was intimidated. This was the man I'd watched in *Rocky* when I was growing up.

"So, uh, how do you feel?" he said.

"I love it," I said. "It's a great project. I'm going to do a good job for you."

"Good, good, all right," he said. "You're my guy."

The next day, the paperwork came in, and it was a go. So I was jumping around from project to project, doing *The Family Crews,* Squeegee, *The Expendables.* I thought I was doing everything it took to succeed. Now I can see I was hypervigilant. I filled my days to feel alive. Well, I was feeling alive then. I was pumped. I really felt like *The Expendables* could be the big one for me.

We started shooting early that spring, and I flew to Brazil. When I got off the plane, I was in for two big surprises. The first one was amazing. I had no idea that *Everybody Hates Chris* was huge in Brazil. Everyone in Hollywood had always told me that black performers only hit in America, and because they couldn't sell us in Europe, or South America, or anywhere else, we weren't worth as much as white performers, and we shouldn't be paid as much. Well, I was so mobbed at the airport that I had to be escorted to a special lounge and wait for security to take me to my car. I couldn't leave the hotel without being mobbed by fans that were waiting for me to come out. But then I decided to see what this was all about. I went running in the streets, and I found that everyone in the country was wonderful. They were so respectful and happy to see me.

The second surprise was not so good. During the month I was in Brazil, I only shot one scene. My character seemed to diminish before my very eyes. Normally, this would have been the kind of development that would have made my insecurities flare up and caused me to act out, as I had on my first film set in Vancouver, a decade earlier. This time, I vowed to behave, and I was lucky enough to have a wonderful tour guide. I threw myself into exploring the beautiful country. I was relieved when shooting in Brazil was over, and I had no more dark secrets to protect, as I was still terrified Rebecca would someday find out what I had done in Vancouver.

I still had to get through the rest of the *Expendables* shoot, and the situation wasn't looking to improve anytime soon. It took only a week on location in New Orleans for me to be extremely disappointed. All of my scenes had either been cut down significantly or cut out completely. I felt like a glorified background player. I was determined to make the most of the situation, even talk to Sly about a potential spinoff, but it was difficult for me not to become cynical, especially when a month went by and I'd spent most of my time sitting in my hotel room.

The project had been poisoned for me. When I went to the set, I saw everything as a negative. If Sly was talking to Jason, I became jealous. When I saw other people exchanging looks on set, I assumed they were talking negatively about me. I hated feeling that way, and I knew I had to reframe it.

It was hard. It was really hard, but this is what I did. Anytime I was given an opportunity I took full advantage of it. When Sly gave me a line, I put everything into it. EVERY-THING. I worked harder, stayed later, and improved my attitude. Slowly, Sly started noticing me. By the middle of June, I began winning Sly over. After we filmed a scene, and everybody else had moved on to the next scene, Sly sat with me and went over every nuance, how to act, and what I should do every moment in front of the camera. He basically taught me how to be an action star.

"When you get your moment, play it to the camera," he said. "Don't turn your head. Don't shrink back in those moments. Carry the ball when you get it."

He pointed out the scenes were I wasn't focused, and the ones in which I was really shining. "Look, you can see it in your eyes," he said.

"That's the detail that I needed to see," I said.

When my attitude improved, my performance did, too, and he let me know.

"Man, you're doing it," he said. "You're staying in shape. Every time I give you a line to say, you're killing it. I've got to tell you, you're really making me happy."

Just like I'd created a net-negative vortex before, when I'd become consumed by my negativity and insecurity, now I created a net-positive vortex. It literally started in my heart, and grew until that was one of the best experiences of my life.

I decided to reframe the *Expendables* experience like I did my security job. I told myself to see the good in everything and everyone around me and not to give off any bad vibes. It worked. Almost instantly, I saw Sly in a new light, and I began to notice things I hadn't before. I watched him shoot for twelve hours, running around like a wild man at sixty-three years old. I realized this film was his baby. He was taking out scenes that didn't work, as he knew the action fans didn't want their heroes pontificating about social injustice. They wanted action, and we were going to give it to them.

Everything started to turn around. We found out that *The Family Crews* had been picked up. Rebecca and the kids came to visit the *Expendables* set in New Orleans. She ran into Sly while she was walking around by the trailers, and he let her in on a little secret, which she ran back to tell me as fast as she could.

"Terry, oh my God, you won't believe this," she said. "Sly just said, 'Your husband has been so amazing, I'm rewriting the script so he saves my life.'"

I couldn't even speak. I just stood there and stared at her, so happy.

"Terry, I can't believe what's happening," she said.

This was one of the moments when Rebecca got excited, and I knew things were really starting to happen, because she's always had an excellent ability to read people and situations (not that I always listened to her, of course; again, that's why this book has a before and an after).

"Terry, this is the one," she said. "When I heard him telling me how good you are, I knew."

By the end of that shoot, Sly was sending dailies to my room and giving me lessons every day on how to make an action movie and how to be an action star. I felt like I was in a dream, because I couldn't believe how good it was after it had first been so bad, one of the worst experiences of my acting career. That was such an important moment for me, because I learned that I truly have the power to reframe anything. Every experience I have in my life begins in my head, and it's up to me to be positive, and learn, and grow, and make it all worthwhile.

I started to see how *Rocky* and *Rambo* got made. Sly was in his sixties, and he nearly killed himself during that shoot, but he wouldn't give up, even when he was limping around the set, and we were running out of time, and people had to leave.

"Sly, I'm with you one hundred percent," I said. "I'm with you. If I have to stay over, I'll do it. Man, I'm here for you."

He appreciated that, and to this day, Sly is not only one of my mentors, but he's also a true, true friend. He's become my biggest champion, and he enjoys everything I've done since then. There's nothing better than hearing him say: "It was really good, man. You've got that comic timing, brother. You go do it."

I think everybody needs a dad, wherever they are in life, someone who can give you a thumbs-up, and in Hollywood, more so than anyone else, Sly Stallone has been that person for me. He's really been a pop to me in the entertainment industry.

He even took my side when I wanted to pull what I saw as a great publicity stunt during the promo tour for *The Expendables,* even though the folks at Lionsgate weren't so sure. We were down on the floor of the New York Stock Exchange, and we'd just rung the opening bell. Now I had something even bigger planned, but the producers had said, "No." And then Sly gave me the bump.

"Hey, man, it's time," he said.

I took off my shirt, and I screamed as loud as I could. The place was like a locker room to begin with, all guys, running around with ticker tape, and the whole place froze. And then everyone laughed and cheered, and the cameras all just went off. At that moment, *The Expendables* was the number-one movie in America, and when that picture hit the wire, it was huge. Well, after that, we were number one again for the next week, and that experience taught me so much about publicity. I had already done the Old Spice ads at that point, and they'd been massive, but this moment was different. I'd learned that beyond playing a particular part, I could sell a project.

"You did good," Sly said. "This is how you do it. You are a real star, man."

To have Sylvester Stallone call me a star, it was beyond belief. Here I was, this kid from Flint, Michigan, and now I was in his inner circle. It was the tops.

Things were rolling. That summer, we finished shooting for *The Family Crews,* and Rebecca had a ball. She was charismatic. She was sweet. She was wonderful. And best of all, she'd started talking the year before about how she wanted to do something huge for our twentieth anniversary. She wanted to have a big party, but I just didn't see where I was going to get that kind of money. I was getting more regular work, but I was still a working actor, and we had five kids. Well, BET decided to kick off the whole show with our twentieth anniversary, and so they paid for our twentieth-anniversary party. We had a huge shindig in Malibu. I used money from the show to get Rebecca a new ring, and it was almost like she had willed it to happen. I danced with her and thought back to our first dance on our first date, when I was just a nineteen-year-old kid with big dreams: *Isn't this crazy?*

E VERYTHING WAS GREAT, AND THEN I HAD TO GO TO CONnecticut in October to start filming *Are We There Yet?* Things got bad, and they got bad really fast. Rebecca didn't want to move. The kids didn't want to move. This was my first star turn, but from the beginning it wasn't turning out as well as I'd hoped. And so, being the controller I was, I tried to make everything better than it was possible to be. I went way beyond what was appropriate in terms of my sense of responsibility for my costars, and the show itself, and this put even more pressure on Rebecca and me.

We were coming up on the premiere of *The Family Crews,* which meant doing press together as a happy family, and yet we were getting along worse than we had in years. And then Rebecca sensed that something deeper was wrong between us.

"Terry, you've done something, and now you're going to put me out here on TV in front of everybody," she said. "I want to know what it was before anything goes down. I don't want any surprises."

I denied it, of course, but I'd never told her what had happened in Vancouver ten years earlier, and I knew she was right: It wasn't fair. *If you don't tell her now, you'll never tell her, and your marriage will never be able to survive this moment.*

More than ever, I was terrified of losing her. I denied and denied. But she could sense there was something I wasn't telling her, and she kept bringing it up.

"I don't want to be somewhere, and somebody comes up and tells me something about you, and I'm going, 'What?'" she said.

And I knew that, with what I'd done, this was a distinct possibility. *Who's to say that it wouldn't happen? Oh my God, that could happen,* I thought.

I knew I had to be fair to Rebecca, but at the same time, it was easy for me to keep making excuses as to why my behavior and my secrecy were justifiable. First of all, I honestly felt like everybody looked at pornography and behaved the way I had. You couldn't have convinced me that everybody didn't have secrets. I'd seen it growing up in my church. I'd certainly seen it in the NFL. Even our former president, Bill Clinton, had been getting up to all kinds of stuff behind closed doors.

I was always comparing myself to people who were a lot worse than I was, in order to make myself feel better. I might have messed up, once, but I didn't have any chicks on the side. And other guys fed into this by telling me I was one of the good guys because I didn't cheat. I'd even gotten a little bit of a strut about this.

MEANWHILE, THERE WERE WARNING SIGNS FROM THE beginning about *Are We There Yet?* I hadn't been given a producer credit. I'd been strong-armed into working with Ali LeRoi again, even though we'd had such issues on *Everybody Hates Chris*. I'd been told I had to go to Connecticut. Once there, we were shooting three episodes a week, which was almost like ending up on the line back in Flint after all, only we were making entertainment instead of cars. This whole time, everyone just kept telling me that once we got the first ten episodes done, we'd get our order for the full 100, and I'd be all set, and so I just had to hang on.

I thought back to *The Expendables,* and I told myself I needed to reframe my experience once again. But instead of just working on my attitude, I took it upon myself to be the pleaser I'd always been, and to be the savior of everyone else on the show. I took a pro-sports mentality, like: If I go out there, and go full speed, and get knocked out on the field, then I'll just get knocked out. Well, usually in the end, you're the guy in the hospital, and they keep on going without you. They love guys like me, who can't say no, who don't have any boundaries.

And so I just kept giving. That's what eventually led to the worst day of my life: D-day. In February 2010, I was working on my new show, and I went to New York City for the weekend. I took my costar out to dinner, trying to act like the producer who was going to fix everything, when there was really no reason for me to do it. I felt like I was responsible for everyone's happiness, and so I didn't realize I was creating more problems than I solved.

Rebecca was still on me about the secret she suspected. "Terry, there's something you're not telling me," she said. "I don't know what it is about you."

"Nah, it's cool."

This went on, over the phone, all night. Meanwhile, a huge snowstorm was bearing down on the city, and even though I was staying at one of the most beautiful hotels, the Mercer, my room was like a prison. It was dark, heavy with snow. All of a sudden, something told me: *Man, this is your opportunity. If you don't tell her now, you're going to be divorced. You're not truthful. You're probably going to lose her if you do tell her, but at least this is a chance for you to actually be clean.*

I really didn't want to tell her. The whole reason I hadn't said anything to her for all of those years was because I knew I was going to lose her if I did. But it kept coming to me: *You've got to tell her. She's got to know who you really are. Everything.*

By morning, the snow had covered up the windows. I felt awful, oppressed, stuck in this dark, dark place. Rebecca called me again.

"Terry, you need to tell me, because you're not telling the truth."

This went on and on. I denied and denied. And then, it just flew out.

"One time, ten years ago in Vancouver, I got a hand job at a massage parlor."

She made a sound that was like a whimper. It was just so much pain. I honestly felt like I'd shot her in the chest. I couldn't believe how much it hurt: It hurt her AND it hurt me. We sat there on the phone, and she just cried and cried.

"How could you do that? How could you even?"

"It was ten years ago."

"That makes it worse. So you've been faking for this long, for ten years?"

I didn't have anything to say in my defense. It really was D-day.

"You can't live here," she said. "You'd better find a place to live. I'm done."

"I know. I know."

I didn't know what to do. It was so dark.

"You put me on television, and you did this, and you never told me."

I understood everything now. I was like: *Oh my God, you're right.* Finally, after another hour on the phone, there was really nothing more to be said, and we hung up. I was lost. I called my current pastor and told him everything.

"Man, what do I do? I'm going to lose her. I wasn't truthful."

"Look, do the normal routine, at the very least," he said. "If you were going to go work out, go work out. If you were going to work, go to work. You don't want to just sit in this. You want to do your normal routine so you don't disintegrate."

So I went, I worked out, I came back. I just tried to hang on. I knew without a doubt I had just lost everything. I was officially done. I was never honest with my wife, or myself. I was broken. For days, I didn't hear a single word from Rebecca.

CHAPTER 17

I'M NOT LIKE THEM

BEGGED AND BEGGED REBECCA FOR HER FORGIVENESS, but she let me sit with what I'd done for several days. Finally, just as I was headed back up to Stamford to start shooting the show again, she called. My heart was pounding.

"Terry, listen, I want to work it out," she said. "I love you, and I forgive you, but I don't know. I don't think anything will ever be the same."

"I know. I know."

"God told me to let you come home," she said.

I was so incredibly grateful. I had really believed I was going to lose her forever, but she'd given me a second chance. It was a miracle. I didn't deserve her. I had hurt her so badly. I couldn't believe the goodness of God.

"One of the requirements for you to even get back into the

house is that you have to get some help about whatever this is," she said.

And then I actually started telling her about the pornography. She didn't know. Nobody knew, not even my best friends knew. I couldn't believe I was getting another chance. But I knew, now the work started.

When I flew home for the first time after D-day, I was nervous as I walked through the front door. All I could think was: *I thought I'd never see this place again. I thought I'd lost all of this, and the ability to even come home.*

The kids ran up to me, and I was so glad to see them, but as I hugged them, all I could do was look at Rebecca. She was crying. We sat down right there in the foyer, before we even got all of the way into the house, and we hugged for a long time. Neither of us said much. She was very quiet. The kids could clearly feel something was up, but they weren't sure what. Again, I thought: *I was sure, after what I'd done, I'd be visiting my kids from here on out.* It was such a relief to be back in that house. It was like being born again, like waking up out of a coma. *I'm still here. I'm not dead.*

Rebecca and I went right up to the bedroom, and we talked, and we talked. She had told me that she had forgiven me, but her anger was still coming out, and it kept flaring up suddenly. She had questions about every little detail of what had happened, and I felt like I had to answer all of them.

After the kids went to sleep, we stayed up talking all night. There were many nights during that time when there was no sleep. Her emotions seemed to attack her at the end of the day. We lay down to go to bed, but she couldn't sleep, and she wanted to talk for hours. There were many nights when I went into the bathroom and found her sitting there crying. I didn't know what else to say. In fact, I knew there was nothing else to say. I usually tried to get in several naps during the day, so I could stay up with her at night while she went through all of this.

During the day, I found her all over the house, just sitting there, crying, and it reminded me of her breakdown following her second miscarriage. I started to worry that this type of stress might take her back into that kind of depression again. In some ways it did; her behavior was so all over the place. I understood why, and I knew I just had to take it, take the anger, take the emotion, and let her have her say.

On top of everything else, the *Family Crews* premiere was nearly upon us, and we were already doing press, trying to act like we were still a big, happy family.

"You put me on TV when you knew what you'd done," she said. "And I did it. We filmed it. What were you thinking?"

I could understand why she felt hurt and betrayed. I just didn't know how to make it better. I reached a point where I was tired of the secrets, tired of being worried it would all come out, and I just started talking about everything to everyone in our life. One night, Rebecca and I went out to dinner with another celebrity couple that had been having their own problems. We sat there at the restaurant, dodging the real issues, and then something inside of me snapped.

I'm not hiding anything anymore, I thought.

I told them exactly what I had done and what we were going through. Well, they both looked at me as if a lizard had just come out of my mouth. They could not understand why I was telling them this. That was not the celeb way to do things.

Oh, boy, I guess that was a mistake, I thought.

But it wasn't long after that they were divorced. So much for the celebrity way.

The next time I saw the husband, he brought it up right away.

"What are you doing, man?" he said. "Why did you tell your wife?"

"Dude, I had to be honest. I had to be real."

"Man, never," he said. "What is your problem? That's man code, brother. You don't tell."

"Well, if that's man code, I'm not a man, then, because I'm not living that way anymore," I said. "I can't do it. How could I be a man if I lived that way?"

As much as I had clung to my fear of telling Rebecca the truth and tried to pretend it was the best thing for both of us, I'd always known, deep down inside, that it was either tell her the truth, or we would just break up later anyhow. You can't build a relationship on secrets and lies. It's not a real, firm foundation. And somewhere inside, she always knew I was keeping something from her. She always suspected something was up. So she would have just kept asking me again, and again, and again, until her questions were finally, really answered.

Rebecca had not forgotten her requirement that I get professional help, and on March 14, 2010, I entered a one-week program that dealt with sex addiction at a place called Psychological Counseling Services in Phoenix, Arizona.

I was willing to do whatever it took to save my marriage, but I was clear on one thing as I checked in and got settled on my first night: *This is crazy. I'm not like them. Maybe I went too far, and it got me here, but that's it. Come on, who doesn't look at pornography? What kind of a man doesn't look at pornography?*

And then, as I talked to my counselors and went to the group sessions, I began to see that there are many people who don't have compulsive behaviors around pornography. There are many people who don't have this problem. From there, it was just one epiphany after another for an entire week.

Early on, I was in therapy, talking with my doctor about my acting career.

"With my job, people ask me to do certain things, and I have to do them."

"Why?"

"Because it's my job."

"But you don't have to do it."

"Yes, I do, because it's my job."

"Get another job."

"But I can't get another job," I said. "This is what I want to do."

"So you want to do it?"

"No, I have to do it."

"No, no, no, you don't have to do anything," she said.

That's a Jedi mind trick, I thought. *Stop it. You're freaking me out.*

"Terry, you always have a choice," she said, smiling at me warmly. "The only reason you feel trapped is because you thoroughly believe you have no choice, but you always have a choice."

In my head, I had no choice about anything. This went back to when I was little, and I really didn't have a choice. But now I was an adult, and maybe she was right. It seeped in slowly, like water through a rock: We always have a choice, every minute of our lives. *Oh my God, I do have a choice,* I thought. *I can say no.*

Up until then, I had really felt like I couldn't say no, to certain opportunities, or to certain requests from directors or fans. Even as I started to believe her, I couldn't imagine a producer telling me to do something, and then me saying NO.

"I feel like I would lose my job," I said.

"First of all, if you lose your job then that's not the job you wanted anyway," she said. "There's always another way to do something. If you feel uncomfortable, you should be able to tell them you feel uncomfortable."

"But how?"

And then it hit me: *Almost all actors are like this. We don't ever say no.*

"All of these actors need to be in therapy," I said.

She watched this new idea dawn on me, and she laughed, not unkindly.

"You're right," she said. "And half of them are."

I laughed, too. It was a funny moment. But it was also a whole new world. *Okay, I have to start saying no. I can say no now.*

I knew what I had to do, but let's just say I had a bit of a learning curve. When I first got home from Phoenix, I stopped at a gas station, and a male fan approached.

"Can I get a picture?" he said.

I immediately went into default mode: *I don't really feel like it, but I don't want to make him mad, or make him not like me, so I guess I should just . . . NO.*

"No," I said.

I had found the word, but my voice was quiet and squeaky. I had to practice.

"No," I said, louder this time. "I'm getting gas."

"Come on, man," he said. "Come on."

"NO," I practically shouted, getting into it now. "NO. NO."

Once I started saying no, after all of those years of being the pleaser and going against my own wishes just to make everyone else happy, it felt so good to say no that I couldn't stop. That poor guy, he got the brunt of all of my therapy, and he didn't even know what he was walking into. He had no clue.

"No, I'm just pumping my gas," I said. "I don't have to give you a picture. I don't owe you anything."

"Dude, get you, man," he said. "I never wanted it anyway."

When he finally walked away, I was still pumping my gas, and as I looked around to see if anyone else had noticed what had just happened, I realized I was shaking. I had never told anyone NO before. And then, suddenly, I felt so light, full of possibility. I didn't have to do things I didn't want to do. It was a whole new world.

After my initial breakthrough, I had a hunger for therapy, and to learn everything I could about human nature in order to understand myself better. I read everything I could put my hands on, books about addiction, psychology, neuroscience, how the brain works, anything to try to figure out what was happening with me, and how I had come to end up in the circumstances I had. Now that I'd experienced such a profound breakthrough, I was embarrassed by my previous ignorance. I could see how arrogant and self-centered I had been, how unconscious I'd been of the forces that drove my thinking and behavior, all the while assuming I knew better than everyone else did. The most horrible moment for me was finally getting that I hadn't known anything before, and I'd even been ignorant of my own ignorance. I didn't ever want to be in that position again, where I didn't know what I didn't know, and I vowed I never would be.

I had another breakthrough during this time. I had started down this path to save my marriage, and I wanted more than ever to be a good husband and father, but I wasn't doing this for Rebecca anymore. I was doing it for myself. And it was perhaps the first unselfish thing I'd ever done in my life. I was taking care of myself so I could be there for my family. And I wanted Rebecca to take care of herself first, too, no matter what it meant for her marriage to me. It was a profound shift, and it wasn't always a smooth process. There were moments when I was still desperately afraid that I was about to lose everything.

I had seen so many other couples fall apart, even ones who'd gone through all of the same kind of therapy as Rebecca and me. And there were times when all I could do was pray. There were moments when it wasn't about how much I was learning or growing, or what technique I was using to be a better person. All it was about was how I didn't want my wife to leave me, and all I could do was fall down on my knees and pray. Sometimes that was all that was left, and it comforted me.

Once Rebecca and I had stabilized things in our relationship to the point where we could live in the same house together, we knew we had to talk to the kids about what was happening. Obviously they'd noticed the tears and tension, and I knew the worst outcome would have been for them to blame themselves in any way. Having grown up in a family where there were many dark truths that were never discussed, and having seen how my own personality was shaped by this environment, I've always felt like we're so backward in choosing to remain silent because we think our kids are too young to understand adult problems, rather than just letting them know that what's happening is not their fault.

Our older two kids could understand a little more, and so I told them a quick version of what had happened without too many details. I sat the younger three kids down together, and I chose my words very carefully.

"Daddy did something that hurt Mommy a lot," I said. "It was outside of our marriage, and it should have never been done, and Daddy didn't say it for a long time. But now Daddy is sorry, and I want to make it better."

They didn't seem all that surprised. What I had learned in therapy, and through my reading, was that the kids already knew something was wrong, and if I hadn't told them, they would have thought it was them. So they seemed relieved, especially after I made sure they knew I wasn't going anywhere.

I continued to be on a quest to understand myself better, and I expanded the range of the material I was reading and listening to as audiobooks. I took in all of the stuff I could absorb about how to be a better husband, how to be a better father. As I did, I was struck by something. As men, we will study how to be the best architect, the best football player, the best actor. We'll spend all the time we can find on our careers. But we need to be spending more time studying how to be a great husband, how to be a great father, how to be a great man.

The more I learned, the deeper my realizations went. I began to understand why I had always messed up financially. And I don't mean I was learning about financial planning, although I definitely came to understand money better, too. I finally grasped the psychological underpinnings for my behavior. Every time I was sad, I needed to get happy, so I spent money. Or I made ridiculous, impulsive decisions, just because I was trying to improve my state of mind, when not spending—and actually saving my money—would give me all I needed in the long run, and forever. I even made risky moves because it was exciting, and I got energized from the risk, which distracted me from feeling bad.

No matter what, I couldn't let myself be sad. Once I realized I needed to experience happiness and sadness, I started to wake up. I realized I also needed to understand empathy. I needed to let myself stop and feel bad for other people, and really listen, and really feel what they were talking about. This started with my family, and my friends, and it expanded to everyone I worked with, and then everyone I encountered every day. It changed the way I thought about everything. EVERYTHING.

I even started to understand the people who cut me off while driving.

Mostly, I came to understand myself. I was forced to see who I really was. I finally realized I'd been so driven over these many years, mostly because of my dark secret, first about the drinking and abuse in my house, and then about my own pornography addiction. Because I always felt dirty, I was basically trying to clean myself by achieving perfection. I made up for my dark secrets by working harder, working longer, working more, getting more fit, perfecting my artistic ability. I had to be that perfect person. I had to be what everybody wanted me to be.

That's how, all of my life, I came to be the primo yes man. If anybody wanted me to do something, I did it. When the coaches asked who was going to do something, I always raised my hand. As an adult child of an alcoholic, I was a pleaser, and as a perfectionist, I was the main pleaser. All my life, I just wanted peace. And so if I felt like I could bring peace to a situation by saying yes to something, I did it. I never really shared what I wanted. And then, when I became a parent, I put this on my kids. I wanted my kids to be that way, too. It had always been my job to do what other people said. And now it was their job to do what I said. Let me tell you, there's discipline, and then there's being a tyrant. I was a tyrant. And when I could finally see all of this, I understood why I'd had tension with my children for years.

I'd made myself into the superhero I'd longed to be as a kid, and it had been hell on my family and friends, and, worst of all, on myself. Coming out of therapy, I had to realize that my attempts to be a superhero had actually hurt me, not made me stronger. Because I was not superhuman; I was just a human, and my attempts to be this superman, this Teflon star, someone infallible who everyone could look at as the perfect man, were eventually my downfall.

Of course, I still write down my goals. I still see the value in being fit and doing my job well. But trying to be perfect will leave you empty-handed, whereas trying to do your best will keep you fulfilled. The best you can do is always good. I realized you don't have to be perfect, you just have to be faithful in your attempts.

Ever since Rebecca and I went through D-day, my focus has been all about rebuilding from the ground up, and not only our marriage, but also the man I am.

Most of 2010 was devoted to righting circumstances at home and finishing up my commitment to *Are We There Yet?* The show had gone from being a strain to becoming almost unbearable. Rebecca had come to associate it with our marital woes, simply because we had been apart on D-day because of my obligations to the show. Not to mention that the stress of shooting three episodes a week during such a chaotic moment in my personal life was a substantial challenge. At the same time, we shot a second season of *The Family Crews.* It was a lot to manage.

In 2011, I flew to Bulgaria to shoot *The Expendables* 2. At first, we had thought about having Rebecca come visit me on the set. Given everything we'd just been through, she was understandably nervous about having me away from home for so long. But I decided, instead, to use our time apart to do what in therapy circles is commonly referred to as a reset. It involved going ninety days without any sexual activity whatsoever. The year before, Rebecca and I had tried it, and we'd lasted seventy days before I broke down. Ever since then, I'd really wanted to complete the exercise, and I knew this was our chance. So we had a ninety-day fast.

The reset began on October 1, and it went all the way to the New Year, even after I returned home to Los Angeles in early December. It was probably one of the best things I've ever done in my life. I didn't realize until then that, as men, we see our wives as sexual beings, and sometimes this means we don't see them as people, or value them as real human beings beyond the bedroom.

At this point, Rebecca and I had been married for twenty-two years, and yet I found we still had so much to discover about each other. It was almost like a courting period all over again. We had long talks, and I came to know her in a deeper way, and to love her even more.

It was another major epiphany for me when I realized I didn't need sex for intimacy, and I didn't need sex to be happy. I started to see how it was possible to take the physical act out of the equation but still be very close. I started to understand all of the ways that sex had become so loaded for me. When I was stressed out, I wanted sex to make me feel better. It had become a way of acting out and relieving stress. I started to look at my relationship with Rebecca differently. Like many men, I'd always believed it was my wife's responsibility to give me sex when I wanted it. But, no, her responsibility was to be intimate, and then, out of that, sometimes, sex will happen. And my responsibility was to be close to her, and to be her sounding board, that one person she could really trust. After twenty-two years, it was like a whole new marriage, and it was blowing my mind.

Ever since then, I break it down for my kids as such: "You're going to leave home someday. But I'm closer to my wife than I am to you, and I made you."

Through all of this, I've come to realize that closeness is not about physical commonality. It's really about the connection you forge. When a person knows everything about you, and she still loves you, that's the closest you can be to another human. And for years, Rebecca and I had always been held back as a couple because of my secrets and the part of myself I was hiding from her. We'd lasted for years, sure, but by the time of D-day, we had finally run out of steam.

And it wasn't until I came clean that I realized what marriage really is. Until your relationship gets to the point where you can tell that other person everything about who you are, everything about what you've done, everything, it can never reach a level of real, true intimacy. Now, you might be stuck together, you might stay together by choice, and it might be okay, but it'll never be great. And it wasn't until after D-day, and until after our ninety days of celibacy, that we finally were closer than we'd ever been. It was like a real lasting breakthrough had happened.

Now, none of this was a cure-all. I could create an amazing relationship with my wife in the present, but I couldn't undo the past. After what I'd done, and what I'd hidden for all of those years, Rebecca didn't trust me, and for good reason. In early 2012, she asked me to take a lie detector test, and I was glad to do it. Not that I enjoyed the process; I had all of the usual fears that the test would go wrong and make it seem like I was lying when I wasn't. But I passed with flying colors, and I was ready to take such a test once a year for the rest of our marriage, if that was what it would take to put her at ease.

CHAPTER 18

MANHOOD

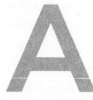S I CONTINUED TO LEARN ABOUT MYSELF, I started apologizing for small mistakes I'd made over the years. And I remained hungry to learn even more. One day, just for fun, I took an online test about narcissism. Well, I was shocked by the results. It said I was a narcissist. I couldn't believe it was true. I went downstairs right away and strode into the living room, where Rebecca was hanging out with the younger kids.

"I just took this online test and it said I'm a narcissist," I said.

"You think?" Rebecca said.

The kids all laughed. Not meanly, but in this kind of sweet way, like they were watching a baby deer learn to walk by falling down every few steps.

I thought back to how I'd made Rebecca trade in the car she liked for one I just knew was better for her. Looking back, I realized that she'd never really liked that new car because she'd never really wanted that new car. She'd liked the one she had better than the one I'd chosen. But I'd picked it out for her, and told her it was what she should drive, without ever asking her what she wanted. I'd thought nothing about just going out and being totally responsible for her. And not just about the car, about meals, about vacations, about everything. I'd always made all of the decisions and expected my family to like it because it was what I wanted.

Ugh, I get embarrassed just thinking about it. Let's just say I apologized a lot during that time, and I'm still apologizing today.

It was a moment of big personal and professional change. We reached the end of *Are We There Yet?* I had worked really hard on that show, even during extremely difficult circumstances at home, and I didn't feel like it was anything more than a moneymaker for many of the people involved. And then they just stopped airing it, mid-season. I was upset, but overall, it was a relief to be done with that arduous period in my life.

We'd come to really love living in Connecticut, and we were thinking about relocating there permanently, when I got the chance to audition for Aaron Sorkin's new TV show, *The News-room.* Everything about that show, from the audition through the filming process, was hard. Even though it was set in New York City, they filmed in Los Angeles, and so when I finally got the part, I had to relocate in advance of my family, while earning almost no money, to do a part that required extreme precision at all moments. And I loved every minute of it. I knew it would only make me better as an actor, which it did. And it was an extreme pleasure to work with people who were so completely devoted to making great art. I'd found my kind of people, and I wanted more of that all of the time.

Through *The Newsroom,* I had the chance to do *Arrested De-*

velopment, which was a similar experience. I also pushed myself physically that year on the reality show *Stars Earn Stripes,* and I broke into new territory with my first voiceover job on the animated feature *Cloudy with a Chance of Meatballs 2.*

The whole family was back in Los Angeles, and it finally felt like we were coming out on the other side of what had been a very difficult time for us all. But I still felt like I was looking for that next project that would continue to push me to grow as an actor, and to take my career to all-new places.

In early 2013, I was actually offered three different pilots because of my work on *The Newsroom* and *Arrested Development.* After my experience on those shows, I was all about whatever would be the best experience creatively. One of the shows was an Andy Samberg project. I'd never met Andy, but I'd always been a fan, and I really felt like he was the future of comedy. I had a meeting with the show's creators, Dan Goor and Mike Schur, who'd also created *Parks and Recreation.* I wasn't sure what show I was going to choose, and then Dan and Mike kept calling me. That wasn't unheard of, but there was something special about their calls.

"We named the character after you," Dan said. "You have an advantage in negotiations now because whoever does take this role is going to be named Terry."

I just laughed when I heard that. I loved their energy, and I knew the show would be a great ensemble. This was what I felt like I needed right then, so I could learn and get better by working with talented people, rather than just wanting to be the star, which, like the attempt to be a superhero or to achieve perfection, is just not a worthwhile goal. I realized that I'd actually learned this long ago, from football. When someone was always hogging the ball, or the spotlight, maybe they were seen as the star, but it backfired on them. In the end, it was the team guys who were really appreciated the most. I wanted to be that dude, that team player, and I felt a show like *Brooklyn Nine-Nine* was the show that would give me that opportunity. It went back even further for me, too, back to *The Carol Burnett Show,* and those great TV ensembles. And so I signed on with *Brooklyn Nine-Nine* in the middle of 2013. Well, all I can say is it's been an absolute pleasure from the beginning, and then to have it be received so well has just been the ultimate reward. So well received, in fact, that in January 2014, we won the Golden Globe Award for Best Comedy from the Hollywood Foreign Press. As I stood on that stage with the rest of the cast, looking over the Beverly Hilton ballroom into the faces of U2, Michael Douglas, Meryl Streep, and Leonardo DiCaprio—all I could feel was thankfulness.

In addition to working harder to be an even better actor and comedian, I now value, more than anything else, the work I've done to become a better man. Once I began to have compassion for myself, and my family, and everyone I encounter, it changed everything. I've learned to validate another person's feelings, and validate who they are, without losing anything of myself or letting my boundaries be compromised. And it has changed literally everything for me: my relationships, my health, my strength, and my life.

I realized that I'd been so lacking in compassion, I hadn't ever shown it to my family before. I'd judged them and condemned them, because I was so hard on myself, and I thought it should be the same for them. But now I can see how wrong that behavior was. Like I said, I've apologized so many times and reminded them that it's still a work in progress.

I can't tell you how happy I am that it wasn't too late to change and be forgiven. Many men have lost their wives and families because they weren't willing to really look at themselves

and take responsibility for their beliefs and their actions. Instead, they went and found a new wife, and a new family, thinking it would be better. But the problem wasn't their wife or
family. It never was. They were the problem. But they never
realized it, and so they ended up seventy and alone, like when
I saw my grandfather get slapped in the face by his own
daughter—a lifetime of selfish, ignorant behavior come to roost.
And it was only then, when it was too late, that it finally dawned
on them: *Oh yeah, the problem was me all along.*

For some men, pride will never let them admit they were
wrong. That's why pride is the gift that keeps on taking. And
why I'm here to tell all of the men out there, crack that shell,
even just a little bit, and it will bust wide open. Once you let in
real feelings, and let people get close to the real you, that's where
the good stuff is.

Rebecca has been the best example of strength I've ever seen.
She illustrated the importance of strength founded on compassion, and I'm so grateful to her for her willingness to show me
these qualities in our marriage. She had compassion for me
when there was a real reason to have nothing but anger and
hate. When she gave me another chance, and told me that she
believed in who I am, no matter what I'd done, it broke me
down in the best possible way and allowed me to rebuild a better
man in the place of who I'd been before. Now, that was compassion at work.

I thank God every day that Rebecca made the choice to stay,
because legally, and by every measure with which we judge a
relationship, she had good reason to leave. And the truth is, even
with the many joyous occasions that happened during our first
twenty years of marriage, the marriage she was fighting for in
the aftermath of D-day wasn't anything as deep as the marriage

we have now. I've gotten so much out of this whole experience that I never even knew was possible.

When I look back at the way I was living before, it reminds me of those Godzilla movies I loved when I was a kid. It seems like all of these monsters are coming out of nowhere, destroying Japan, but the truth is, the monsters were there all along, moving around among the people, only they were small enough that everyone ignored them. It wasn't until they became 200 feet tall, and were tearing up buildings, and nearly unstoppable, that the citizens finally had to fight them. And then they were much harder to defeat than they would have been when they were just baby monsters. That's how I came up with the motto by which I now run my life: Destroy All Monsters. I have vowed to never again let my monsters grow so big. My mantra is: *Humble yourself. Discover what your monsters are. Be honest with yourself.*

These changes started with my wife, and they expanded to my children, and I've taken them outward from there into all areas of my life. My old friend Ken and I talk about it all the time. We can laugh about it now, as we recall the path I had to stumble down in order to grow, and how I once got so mad at him for refusing to help me anymore after he'd already given me so much.

"You're going to call your production company Gold Coin Productions," he teased me.

I very well could have, because those gold coins were a symbol of the lifeline he sent out to me, and the moment when I finally had to grow up and start doing for myself, and, really, the first humbling of many I've received to get where I am.

I have since built a tremendous relationship with my mother, as we laid everything out on the table and rebuilt from the ground up. It was hard. Angry words were spoken, and for a while we found it impossible to talk to each other. As time passed I was able to put my anger aside and just love my mother for what she did do for me, rather than being angry for what she didn't. I asked her to forgive me for my sense of entitlement and for holding on to offense, and she asked me to forgive her for any wrong she'd done. I told her I realized she'd done the best she could with what she'd been given, and I'm thankful for her and the beautiful woman she is. My mother was the only one to take care of Mama Z, my grandmother, my grandfather, Sister Estes, and many others before they died. The truth is, I could always count on her, even to this day, and my love for her has no bounds.

From there, my personal growth has expanded to one of the most challenging relationships in my life, my relationship with Big Terry. There were times after the Christmas from Hell when I couldn't bring myself to answer his calls for months at a time. And then something would shift within me, and one day, he'd call, and I'd pick up. But we never seemed to make any real progress, no matter how much we talked.

"Terry, I never had a father to show me how to be one," he said. "I got a lot of pain, and all I tried to do was give you guys better than what I had. I didn't know what else to do. I knew to give you a roof."

I could hear the truth in that. But there were other times when he deluded himself, and I couldn't stand to let him run off at the mouth like that.

"I taught you guys everything you know," he said.

"No, Big T, that's not how it went down," I said.

He paused then, and sat quietly for a minute.

"Yeah, I guess not," he said.

After another pause, he couldn't quietly let it go, though.

"But I did teach you to be your own man," he said.

"Uh, I guess."

In all of these conversations, I always felt dissatisfied. I think I was waiting for him to apologize, to really see how things had been, and talk to me about it. And then it finally hit me that if he was ever really going to get it, the moment of clarity had to start from me. I had to tell him, honestly, what was up. But this wasn't in the way most people would think. As I made myself really look at what had happened all those years ago, I started to see him differently, and then I started to see all of the things I'd been through differently. I'd always looked at my past as this horrible experience that I had to forget, as if it was just a bad feeling that I had to move past.

But no, I needed to sit in it and take those experiences for what they really were. It had been bad, sure, but it had made me who I am. This didn't mean that some of the things that had happened weren't wrong, but they had truly made me stronger, and not just in the fantastical way of superheroes. Life had made me stronger only because I had learned from it. Once I saw Big Terry differently, I was able to identify the aspects of my childhood that I appreciated, which was much different than the way I'd looked back on my past before. Much like I'd done on various sets, and with various work relationships, I reframed my past, and my relationship with my father: *You knew your father. He was at home, and he cared enough about you to clothe you, to feed you. He never beat you. He never left the family. He could have cheated and run off with some girl.*

I started giving Big Terry credit for what he did do. He was a good earner. He was a good provider. I never excused what had been wrong, but also being able to see the positive finally changed my perspective. It changed my view of our story.

Big Terry always felt like he had done better than the previous generation, and I started to see him and appreciate that. I saw that I'd gone even a bit further than he did, and I hope my son will go further than I did someday. He doesn't have to go through all of the different hardships I went through, but he'll have his own struggles, too.

Finally, it all became clear to me, and I called my father.

"Big Terry, I truly believe this, man," I said. "If I could choose who my parents were, I would choose you."

It took a lot to say it, but it was the absolute truth. I realized if I had Bill Cosby as a parent I could have ended up in a whole different place, and not necessarily a good one, either. I've seen great kids come from terrible parents, and I've seen awful kids come from the best parents. And for me, Big Terry and Trish are how I got here.

"I would choose you all over again if I could pick my parents," I said. "I would pick you."

He cried and he cried. And talk about a breakthrough, as soon as those words came out of my mouth, everything changed. He was suddenly humble.

"Terry, I'm sorry for what I did to you and Marcelle," he said. "I was wrong."

WOW. As much as I had longed for an apology from my father for all of those years, I had never really thought it was possible. But by finding my own compassion for him, I had broken down everything that needed to be broken within him. Before that, I'd always hoped that when he got himself together, he'd come to me. I'd always been waiting for him. When, really, he was just waiting for that from me.

"Terry, I want to be better," he said. "I love you, son. I'm proud of you. You did good."

Just those few words from him were exactly what I'd needed to hear to break something open inside of me, and we were able to finally heal. I'm so grateful for that moment. And I really think much of it was only possible because of how I'd witnessed Rebecca handle our marriage. My anger toward Big Terry was perfectly justifiable, just like her anger toward me, but if I'd just stayed in that anger, and in my pride, there would have been no way for the relationship to move forward and to deepen and grow. Once I'd humbled myself, and once I'd had the courage to lead with compassion rather than anger, as I'd seen Rebecca do, I realized that everything is not about good or bad. It's about what you can learn from it.

I don't get the chance to go back home that often, but when I traveled back to Flint in the fall of 2013, I went out to breakfast with my mother, father, and sister. We talked some things out that we hadn't talked about in a long time, and it wasn't acrimonious at all. It was healing, and we were all at peace.

This is what it is, I thought, *never denying things, but just acknowledging them and learning from them, and then leaving them behind to move on with our lives.*

After breakfast, we were out in the parking lot. I hugged Big Terry, and then, as my arms were around him, I wouldn't let him go. I hugged him like I had when I was four years old, really squeezing him tight. For a minute, I felt him tense up, like *okay,* and then he just let go, and I kept holding him, and he let me. I never could have imagined hugging him like that before, and if I'd stayed in my manly sense of my pride, I never would have been able to, either. I think he realized this, too.

He called me the next week.

"That hug you gave me," he said. "That was a good hug. It was wonderful."

R IGHT NOW, I'M ALL ABOUT REVERSING AS MUCH OF THE damage of the past as I can—pain that was caused to me, and pain that I've caused to others. And I've discovered something really amazing along the way, too. As long as it takes to mess something up, it doesn't take nearly as long to fix it. It takes a while to do it right, sure, it definitely takes a while. But I've seen it with my father, and I've seen it with my wife: You can make up twenty-five years of mistakes in five years. If you start healing today, you will gain momentum much more quickly than you think, and even before you're all the way there, you'll feel so much better along the way.

I don't ever want to go back, with Big Terry, or anyone else in my life. I don't ever want to go back to feeling resentful toward people. And I don't want to create any more damage in the future. When I see my kids struggling with the growing pains we all have as we go through life, I try to model compassion and patience.

"Your father's been through a lot of therapy," I say to them. "Your father is not perfect. There were times when I totally blew up. And I'm telling you that I'm not perfect. So how can I expect you to be?"

I'm especially mindful with my son because I know from my own experience how stupid men can be, and how many limiting ideas of masculinity we take on, and the damage they can do in our relationships and in our lives. I know the day is coming when it will be time to talk to him about what it means to be a man. And right now, I'm just working on creating trust and really building our relationship, so he knows he can say anything to me.

I don't want his experience to be like mine was. When I was a young man, I could never get any questions answered. And I want him to know that no question is off-limits or wrong. I want to be able to explain sex and love and life to him without shock or shame. This is how it works. This is what people feel. And this is how women should be treated. You have sisters. You wouldn't like your sister being treated badly, or even looked at like she's an object. Let's talk about what that means for the women you encounter in the world, because that's someone's sister. That's someone's mom. Someone loves them. You have to respect who women are and treat them like human beings, not objects to be ogled and used. Women have feelings, and you do, too, and to deny their feelings is just going to make you feel bad about the man you're becoming.

Well, he's only eight right now. But I'm really looking forward to those talks.

It's funny because my whole life was dedicated to the pursuit of being a superhero, of being stronger, faster, harder, larger than life. For years, I dedicated myself to this, on the football field, and in Hollywood, and I've actually accomplished much of what I set out to do, and so much more. But, as I look back on everything, there is no greater accomplishment for me than this: being present enough to fully enjoy moments like this one.

During the summer of 2013, Rebecca sang the National Anthem at a Los Angeles Dodgers baseball game. And, truly, that experience was better than anything else I've ever done. I was there as a spectator, with all of our kids, all together, and to watch her sing and kill it, and to watch the crowd go nuts, that was literally the best feeling I've had, ever.

I looked over at the kids Rebecca and I have created and loved together.

"Your mommy's living her dream," I said.

I looked out at the field. The sun was setting, and the palm trees were dark against the golden sky where the sun was going down. Rebecca did such a great job, and she was so happy. And being there for her was better than anything else I'd ever done on my own. My blessings were never for me. They were for her, my kids, and anyone else this story of my life touches. And that's the real secret to manhood: having the courage to be man enough to support the ones who make you great.

ACKNOWLEDGMENTS

Rebecca Crews, my children Naomi, Azriel, Tera, Wynfrey, and Isaiah. My granddaughter, Miley, and son-in-law, Jorge. My parents, Terry and Patricia Crews; my brother, Marcelle; my sister, Michaell. Zella Wright (Mama Z), my grandmother Mary Moore, my grandfather General Simpson. My mother-in-law Anna King Lund, my Uncle Buddy Simpson, my Aunt Paulette Simpson Haynie, my cousins A.J. and Monique. My sister-in-law Tramelle, and nieces Charisma and Faith. My grandmother Ermelle Williams (Suk), my Aunt Marketa Moore, my Aunts Faye, Clare, and Bright. The late, great Claude Smart. My Uncle Sonny Crews, Robert Blonde, JoNathan Watkins, Darwin and Andria Hall, Ken and Janice Harvey, Jerome and Muriel Espy, Micheal Lewis, Joe and April Applewhite, Trevor Ziemba, Gary Bruening, Lee Williams, John Davidek, Matt and Vanita Wamble, Ron Croudy, Charles Estes, Jean Estes, Doug and Robin Parker, Ronnie Jones, John Robinson, Bobby Ross, Pastor

Joel Brooks, Al Molde, Orlando Wilson, Pierre Mayo, Don Sparks, Craig Sutters, Derrick Carr, T. K. Kirkland, Reginald Hudlin, Robert Wise, James Gutierrez, Troy Zien, David Krintzman, Brad Slater, Andy McNicol, Steve Perrine, Marnie Cochran, Sarah Tomlinson, The Anderson Group, Eric Fulton, Kelli Miller, Mark Allenbach, Arnold Schwarzenegger, Sylvester Stallone, Eddie Murphy, Adam Sandler, Keenen Ivory Wayans, Shawn and Marlon Wayans, Damon Wayans, Damien Dante Wayans, Craig Wayans, Chris Rock, Ali LeRoi, Owen Smith, Ice Cube, Katt Williams, Dan Goor, Micheal Schur, Andy Samberg, Andre Braugher, Stephanie Beatriz, Melissa Fumero, Joe Lo Truglio, Chelsea Peretti, Joel McKinnon Miller, Dirk Blocker, Antoine Fuqua, Ravi and Michele Mehta, Stephen Brown, Floyd, Lloyd, and Troy Weaver, DeAndre Richmond, Tichina Arnold, Tyler James Williams and family, Tequan Richmond, Imani Hakim, Whoopi Goldberg, Aaron MacGruder, Aaron Sorkin, Pete Segal, Micheal Ewing, Michael Strahan, Eva Longoria, Tony Parker, Ronny Turiaf, Thierry Henry, Chris Daughtry, Charlie Murphy, Charlie "Mack" Alston, Matt and Rick Alvarez, Arsenio Hall, Romeo Bandison, Carl Banks, Buckshot, Ernie Barnes, Robi Reed, D'Angela Proctor, Nia Hill, Matt and Jimmy Blondell, Nana Boateng, Bobby Boyd, Wayne Brady, Eric Brantley, Mark Taylor, Antonio Fargas, Justin Bua, Dale Comstock, Frank Coraci, Kevin Grady, Jason Statham, Randy Couture, Dolph Lundgren, Jet Li, Bruce Willis, Wesley Snipes, Will and Jada Smith, Steve Austin, Jeff Daniels, Mario Van Peebles, Vincent Pastore, Lester Speight, the late Michael Clarke Duncan, Tiny Lister, Tommy Davidson, David Alan Grier, Mike Judge, Victoria Thomas, Daryl Eckman, Rodney Jerkins, Kem, Anthony Hamilton, Bebe Winans, Israel Houghton, Dr. Jim and Marguerite Reeve, Danny Giles, Bill Goldberg, Tracy Gray, Brad Harper, Michael Irvin, Deion

Sanders, Michael Jai White, John Murphy, Dana Jones and family, Dan and Ellen Kolsrud, Mtano Loewi, George Longwell, Fuzzy Kremer, Elic and Natasha Mahone, Arthur and Stephanie Harris, Bart Mandel, Psychological Counseling Services, Curtis Martin, Rusty McClennon, Will Packer, Dr. Clifford Penner, Michael Rooker, Devon Shepard, Shiyena, and Sinbad. Many apologies to any and all I may have failed to acknowledge on this page.

ABOUT THE AUTHOR

TERRY CREWS is a former model (Old Spice) and NFL player (Los Angeles Rams, San Diego Chargers, Washington Redskins, and Philadelphia Eagles). After the NFL he became an actor, and he now has a long list of credits to his name, including work on *The Newsroom, Arrested Development, Everybody Hates Chris,* and in such films as *The Expendables* franchise, *Bridesmaids,* and *The Longest Yard.* He now stars on the Golden Globe Award–winning Fox sitcom *Brooklyn Nine-Nine* and has roles in six movies releasing in 2014. He has been married to musician and inspirational speaker Rebecca Crews for almost twenty-five years. They have four daughters and one son.

ABOUT THE TYPE

This book was set in Granjon, a modern recutting of a typeface produced under the direction of George W. Jones (1860–1942), who based Granjon's design on the letterforms of Claude Garamond (1480–1561). The name was given to the typeface as a tribute to the typographic designer Robert Granjon (1513–89).